TALKING
ABOUT LUPUS

TRIONA HOLDEN

DR GRAHAM HUGHES
Consultant

PIATKUS

First published in Great Britain in 2004 by
Piatkus Books Ltd
5 Windmill Street, London W1T 2JA
email: info@piatkus.co.uk

The moral right of the author has been asserted

A catalogue record for this book is available from the British Library

ISBN 0 7499 2468 3

Edited by Krystyna Mayer
Text design by Goldust Design

Extract from *Blackadder II* reprinted by kind permission of Richard Curtis and Ben Elton. Copyright © 1985

This book has been printed on paper manufactured
with respect for the environment using wood from
managed sustainable resources

Typeset in Bembo by Palimpsest Book Production Limited,
Polmont, Stirlingshire

Printed and bound in Denmark by Nørhaven Paperback A/S, Viborg

This book was made possible thanks to the remarkable team at St Thomas' Hospital and the patients who kindly shared their stories. I would like to especially thank Prof. Ian Palmer whose love and support kept the project – and me – on course.

Contents

PART II

Foreword by Elaine Paige

Lupus is a distressing disease that can have a devastating effect on those who live with it as well as all their loved ones. One of the worst aspects is that there is widespread ignorance about the disease and in my experience this is not just amongst the public but within the medical profession as well. It is remarkable that so few people are aware of this debilitating illness, especially when you consider how common it is – I am told that in the UK alone there are more cases of lupus than MS, ME, HIV and leukaemia put together! Over the years I have met many lupus patients who talk about their struggle to get a diagnosis. It is a terrible experience to have to live with symptoms that cannot be identified. Not to be able to put a name to what is wrong can be a depressing notion. This is why I think it is crucial to raise awareness of this disease. One way of doing this is to produce such a book as Talking about Lupus which comes from the very important perspective of those with lupus, a 'patient's eye view'. After all, who understands the disease better than those who have it?

For about twelve years I have supported the wonderful work of Dr Graham Hughes and his team as patron of the Lupus Trust in St. Thomas' Hospital, London, where international scientists carry out essential research into the disease; now I would like to see awareness of lupus improved dramatically and that is why I want to support this book by Triona Holden.

Elaine Paige

Foreword by Brian Hanner

In 2003 LUPUS UK celebrated 25 years of organised support for people with lupus. The charity now has thousands of members in 30 regional groups and a burgeoning programme of patient support, research funding, better public awareness and further education on lupus for health professionals.

Lupus organisations are increasingly working together internationally and the first World Lupus Day is to be proclaimed in New York during the May Triennial Lupus Congress for doctors and patients. It is therefore timely that Triona Holden, herself a lupus patient, has written this valued book to reach a wide international readership and which will explain as never before the dilemma that is lupus.

I am delighted to be able to commend Triona's book warmly to readers.

Brian Hanner
Director, LUPUS UK

Foreword by Richard Furie

For ages lupus has mystified the medical community. In fact, even in the modern era, unsolved questions abound. In spite of the complexity of this disease, Triona Holden has written a very clear yet comprehensive book. The scientific information is well written and easy to understand, and the vignettes throughout the book are appealing to patients.

This marriage of medical information and patient stories has created a book that contains everything patients and family members need to know about lupus. Using knowledge, experience and expert communication skills Triona Holden has successfully confronted a multifaceted illness and explained it in meaningful terms that all will understand.

Richard Furie, MD
Member, the SLE Foundation Medical Advisory Board
Chief, Division of Rheumatology and Allergy–Clinical
Immunology
North Shore University Hospital, Manhasset, NY

Preface by
Dr Graham Hughes

I suppose I am the wrong person to write this preface. If I were diagnosed with an illness as mysterious and as daunting as lupus, I suspect that my reaction would be that of many physicians – I would bury my head in the sand. I would run away and avoid the library and internet!

Yet with lupus in particular I also know as a physician that this attitude is faulty. There can be few diseases in which knowledge of the condition helps to improve the outcome so much. In the 33 years since I set up Europe's first dedicated lupus clinic, I have seen a sea change in attitude, knowledge and clinical outcome in this disease.

In the 1960s and 1970s lupus was widely considered as rare, even untreatable. The changes have been spectacular. Firstly, lupus is now regarded as a common disease worldwide, outstripping multiple sclerosis, leukaemia and even in some countries rheumatoid arthritis. The outlook has improved beyond measure. One of the main reasons has been education – both of the medical profession and of the public. I have worked for some time with Triona Holden and truly admire both her approach to the disease and her ability to get her message across. Because lupus is, undoubtedly a complex disease, I feel it is important that more accessible books such as this are made available.

For those patients suffering from lupus who are brave enough and wise enough to learn more about their illness, this book will surely help them through a frightening and often lonely time.

Dr Graham Hughes
St Thomas' Hospital

Introduction

Let me start by giving my reasons for writing *Talking About Lupus*. For many years I was a correspondent for the BBC. During the course of my work I reported on numerous conflicts around the world. I was based with an RAF Tornado unit in the first Gulf war, and was one of the first journalists across the border in northern Iraq. I came under heavy artillery fire at the front line during fighting in the Eritrean war for independence against Ethiopia, worked in South Africa during a military coup in Lesothto and in China after the conflict in Tiananmen Square, and was mugged during urban riots in the UK.

On all these occasions I had no time to think about saving my skin – I was too busy worrying about making my deadline and getting my report on air. I also knew that I could leave the fighting behind by simply stepping on a plane and heading home. All that changed when I discovered I was actually fighting my own war and this time there was no easy escape route. This conflict was not against an easily identified enemy like Saddam Hussein. My assailant was much more sinister – I was under fire from within. My own body was attacking itself. It sounds insane, like a science-fiction nightmare, but this was no dream; for me it was a reality that will colour the rest of my life.

I first became ill when I was filming special reports for the main BBC TV News in the orphanages of Romania.

I contracted a virus with flu-like symptoms. Despite the fever I kept working, because we were on a tight schedule and an even tighter budget. The real problems began when I got home from Romania. The first things to be affected were my eyes: it suddenly felt as though a knife had been thrust into my eye sockets and I had difficulty seeing. In the following weeks and months I experienced numbness, which spread across my fingers, toes and lips. Eventually I couldn't breathe without experiencing pain, and found that my exhaustion was so severe that I struggled to get out of bed. My joints ached as though I had done a full workout at the gym, when in fact I had been lying paralysed on the couch all day.

After two years of tests my rheumatology consultant pronounced his verdict. He confirmed that I had a form of connective tissue disease called lupus, an incurable auto-immune condition. You might think my reaction to this was rather odd. I laughed – not for joy or pleasure, but because I felt an almost unbearably sharp feeling of relief and gratitude. I wanted to embrace the consultant, buy him nice things and get him a knighthood at least. If you've ever been ill – I mean ill with a capital 'I' – you will under-stand that moment when you get a diagnosis, when the insanity and uncertainty melt away and are replaced with knowledge and hope. I had a name for my condition at last, and wouldn't have to shrug my shoulders when people asked me what was wrong, or have to haunt the medical sections in bookshops searching through endless publica-tions about symptoms to try and get to the bottom of the mystery. The words had been spoken, wise judgement had been pronounced and with that came a form of liberation; I could prepare to reclaim my life.

The worst thing that can happen to someone who is fiercely independent is to become a captive. The autoimmune disease lupus makes you a prisoner in your own body, embattled and threatened by the mechanism designed to defend you. It's like having a terrorist working inside you. The white blood cells that make up your personal army turn traitor, ganging up on you, working kamikaze-style against your body. Because it comes from within you can't help wondering if you somehow made it happen; if you pressed the trigger. But you didn't. The chances are that your ancestors are to blame – although no one is quite sure of this, there is growing evidence that people have a genetic predisposition to lupus.

From the moment I knew what was wrong I had to know more. The quickest path to information was the Internet. I logged on and began to browse through the findings of doctors and my fellow sufferers all around the world. At first I was surprised to see so much material about a disease that I had never heard of. The first article I read was written by a rheumatologist in New England in the US. It said something along the lines of 'the outlook for lupus patients is much better than it was twenty years ago or more . . . with improved diagnostic techniques and medications these days they can expect to live for up to ten years'. I was aghast. I had two small children and ten years wasn't enough. It meant that I would die before I reached fifty. Middle age suddenly had a pleasant honey-coloured ring to it. No, ten years was not the answer I was looking for. I had never really considered my own death, and although I had been en route to it a few times early on in my illness I had no intention of shuffling off anywhere. So reading those harsh words rattled me to the core.

Fortunately I found my way to the various charity websites in the UK and the US. They showed that our friend in New England was misleading. I was particularly fond of the phrase 'with the right treatment, these days sufferers can expect to live a normal life'. Hope returned. But that brief journey to despair as a result of dated medical articles made me acutely aware of how important it was for people with lupus to have easy access to the most up-to-date information. There is nothing worse than feeling you are utterly in the dark with only a raging immune system to keep you company.

I bought all the books about lupus I could get hold of – it didn't take long as there were so few of them – and they became well-thumbed friends. As new symptoms presented themselves I would turn to my modest library to compare notes and ensure that I wasn't going mad. After a time, however, I felt I needed to know more and wanted to hear from others like me. As I began to write articles about lupus and interview fellow sufferers I realised how comforting and enabling it was to share this nasty disease with people who really understood. How bizarre does it sound to an outsider when you say you get night sweats in the middle of winter; that you wake up soaking with no other symptoms? Yet if you mention this to many lupus sufferers they will nod their heads knowingly and share with you the tricks they have developed to cope with this problem.

Having lupus is like being an involuntary passenger on a massive rollercoaster – one with dramatic ups and downs. I hold on to the hope that the ups will be as extreme as the downs and that if I am lucky I will get large sections on middle ground. I think the greatest factor in getting through this ride is having the right attitude. You have to decide to take control of it, not vice versa. One way of finding strength is through other people. Sharing the burden, even if it's just for a few minutes on the phone or over a cup of tea, can make all the difference.

I will always remember the first woman I interviewed

at the lupus clinic at St Thomas' Hospital in London. She had been terribly ill with a myriad of symptoms. So varied and universal were her problems that no one believed she was really ill. She related how she had lost all her friends because they thought she was attention-seeking when she told them that she was too ill to get out of bed, even though she looked as though she had just got back from a health spa. I recall how she complained that lupus made her look well. That rang a bell with me; I instantly knew what she meant, and it felt so good to share that particularly annoying aspect of this fickle disease. People had often commented to me that I was looking great when inside my body was tearing itself apart. Systemic lupus isn't like any other disease – a feature of it is that it can actually make your skin have what appears to be a healthy glow.

I accept that it is probably better to look well than pale and death-like, but actually looking really healthy when you are devastatingly ill brings with it incredible problems. Imagine that you are at work and lupus is kicking in – will your boss believe that you are at death's door when you look as though you have just got back from a Mediterranean holiday? There is also something utterly frustrating in the psychology related to ill health. Those around you almost feel cheated if they cannot see a tangible impact of this dreadful disease. It's not like a broken leg or Parkinson's disease. I think that is why so many people have difficulty getting a diagnosis. Firstly it is hard to be taken seriously; and secondly they feel ashamed that they don't look ill enough to feel as bad as they do – so they begin to wonder if it is all in their minds.

That's not to say lupus sufferers never look sick. There were episodes for me when my friends and family started to worry. The blood drained from my face and I looked tired. Dark circles appeared under my eyes – as a dear friend from New Zealand puts it, 'Your bags are packed, babe.' At least then the doctors would take one look at me and swing into action without having to ask how I felt. For some people the nasty raised skin rashes are all too obviously an indication that the disease is active.

These past few years of my life have been a painful journey, one that diverted me away from the path I had constructed for myself and onto a completely alien one that was forced upon me. In all that darkness there was tremendous light – the love and support of my children, my family and friends. I also had the good fortune to find myself in the care of some of the best in the business. The result is that I am generally well these days, and when I feel symptoms coming on I know what to do to keep the disease at bay. I got my life back, a little altered but wonderful nonetheless. I am living proof that lupus can be tamed. It was a joy the other day to see my consultant and hear him tell me that I had extremely mild lupus and that I was doing very well.

I am particularly grateful to Dr Hughes of St Thomas' Hospital, who has been an integral part of *Talking About Lupus*. His expertise and ability to communicate information to a non-medical audience has been invaluable at every stage, as has guidance from numerous doctors worldwide who have contributed by sharing their specialist knowledge.

As I look back over these recent years I am beginning to make sense of it all. Writing *Talking About Lupus* is one of the things that has made me come to terms with having lupus in my life. When I began researching material and interviewing other people with lupus, I wondered if I was mad to confront the disease in this way – reading about the young people who had died, hearing about the terrible impact that lupus has had on so many incredible people.

Once I got past the initial fear, however, I decided that the book had to be written – after all, the only two real weapons I have are knowledge and the ability to communicate it. This is the book that I wish I could have had by my side in those early years – one that answers lupus sufferers' questions in a manageable way, minus the medical jargon. I hope you will find in it comfort, support, knowledge and hope, and that it will give you the chance to share the stories of a selection of remarkable people.

Part 1

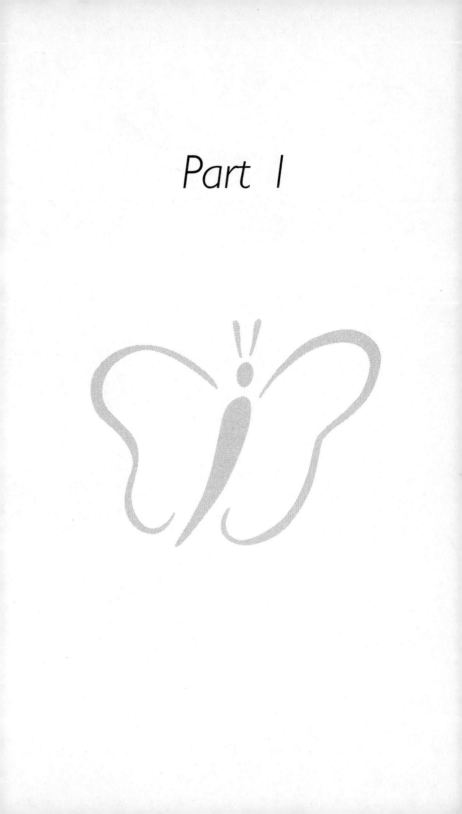

Chapter 1

The Medical Bit

The other day while I was at the checkout queue in a super-market, the woman working at the till was chatting to a customer in front of me about being unwell. She complained that she was exhausted and had joint pains, headaches and mouth ulcers. She'd had a plethora of tests but still didn't know what was wrong and the doctors were stumped by all her symptoms. I am afraid I couldn't resist putting my oar in. 'Perhaps you have a condition known as lupus,' I volunteered. The checkout lady looked horrified 'Oh no – I can't have that,' she exclaimed, almost dropping the box of free-range eggs she was swiping. 'That kills you, doesn't it, and it's contagious. You won't catch anything off me love.'

For me that just about summed up the frustrating lack of awareness of this disease. I did try to put her right. As I unpacked my trolley I gave her chapter and verse about how lupus wasn't a disease that was transmitted from one person to another; how it was treatable and rarely fatal. She just shook her head and got on with checking out my foodstuffs so quickly that they all got crushed at the end of the conveyor belt. I didn't say I had lupus but she obviously suspected as much and wanted to get rid of this disease-ridden customer as quickly as possible.

Ignorance is one of the worst enemies you face when

3

you have lupus. It isn't simply a lack of awareness among the general public – sadly, a disturbing number of doctors are just as guilty of being in the dark about the disease. In fairness, though, this is changing, albeit slowly. These days the growing number of vocal charities and campaigners has helped open people's eyes, but there is still a long way to go. As a patient yourself, or someone close to a person who has lupus, the best thing you can do is educate yourself about the disease. Read the books, log on to the Internet, where there are plenty of excellent sites, talk to other people in the same situation as you and don't be afraid to tackle your GP or specialist about lupus. Knowledge will put you in the driving seat. If you know what symptoms point to this condition and what blood tests or treatments to ask for, you will have the best chance of getting what you want. Doctors generally don't like patients who come armed with mountains of paperwork to support their 'self-diagnosis', but remember that it is your body and therefore you are ultimately the person responsible for ensuring that you get the right care to keep you well. Chapter 12 provides an action plan that gives advice on how to prepare for a consultation so that you can get the most out of it.

'Don't panic'

If you have just been told that you have lupus or suspect as much, *don't panic*. The very fact that the name of the disease has entered your vocabulary is an important first step. Having an identity for your illness helps you to take positive action to deal with it and get it under control. These days the management of lupus has progressed to the extent that the majority of people who are diagnosed and treated can expect to live normal lives. The more tricky cases are those people who have been ill for years without a diagnosis, thereby giving the disease time to do damage to major organs. Fortunately the number of people who fall into this category is mercifully low.

So what is lupus?

Lupus is a highly complex disease, and no one knows what causes it or how to cure it – yet. It is fickle; a flare can come and go for no apparent reason. It can be so mild as to be insignificant, or it can be fatal. The majority of people experience it between the two extremes. Lupus is a bully, hiding in the shadows and striking unseen and often without any warning just when you are feeling at your weakest. Not only does it mimic other conditions and doesn't fit neatly into any medical slots, but also the myriad of symptoms make it hard to define, so that getting a diagnosis can be difficult. The best way to deal with this bully is to expose it – to bring it out into the open. That way you have a much better chance of fighting back. Knowing and understanding lupus are the primary tools you need to get this bully under control. If you take some basic steps towards learning more about the disease you will have a vastly improved chance of getting the better of it.

Lupus is an autoimmune disease. If you look up autoimmune in a medical dictionary you will get the following type of description: 'Autoimmune disorders are where a person's immune system reacts against the organs or tissues of his or her own body. The immune system is there to respond to antigens – invading microorganisms like bacteria or viruses. It produces blood proteins called antibodies and cells known as lymphocytes that will recognise and destroy the antigens. Autoimmune disorders happen when these defence reactions occur against the body's own cells and tissues.'

That's the way a doctor might describe it. A layperson would start by explaining that there are red and white cells in your blood. The white cells function like your own personal army – they are your immune system, there to defend you against invaders from outside, like bacteria or a virus. For instance, if you cut yourself and expose part of your body to external bacteria, the white blood cells rush to the point of injury to fight off the germs. It's nature's brilliant defence mechanism and for most people it is a lifesaver. 'Autoimmune' is when that army becomes confused and overactive – 'auto' meaning 'self'. So the immune system turns against itself and decides to attack rather than protect your body. Because this army of white blood cells has access to all your body any part of it can be affected.

In systemic lupus erythematosus (SLE), the most severe form of the disease (*see page 8*), there is no limit to the areas that can be targeted and no way of guessing where it will strike. SLE is a disease that prompts a plethora of questions to which there are no answers. For instance, no one knows why you get it, how it will manifest itself in each individual or what the outcome is likely to be. It can be so mild that it is virtually symptom free, or it can be so aggressive that it can kill. SLE can target major organs, the nervous system or the connective tissue that holds together the various structures of the body.

The disease affects each person differently, which makes it difficult to summarise how lupus affects people. There are common symptoms, though – lupus sufferers often have one or a number of the following: painful joints, rashes, chronic fatigue, ulcers, hair loss, headaches, depression or behavioural changes, kidney disease, fever or blood disorders. What makes matters worse is that the symptoms can change from one flare to the next in both type and severity. So someone who has had crippling knee and hip pain on one occasion may suffer from rashes and ulcers on another.

To further complicate the picture there are a number of different types of lupus, and it is not uncommon for a person to have other autoimmune conditions at the same time (*see page 54*). You can find yourself the not-so-proud owner of a list of odd-sounding diseases. It is hardly any wonder that doctors have problems getting to the bottom of what is wrong with patients who have so many disparate and changeable symptoms.

I know the idea of the body attacking itself sounds odd. If this was described in a science-fiction novel you would have publishers turning the manuscript down as too unlikely. But there you have it – that is what we are dealing with when it comes to lupus.

As you will read in later chapters, SLE can be fatal, but in the majority of cases the disease can be controlled. The key is getting a diagnosis. In lupus more than in almost any other disease, diagnosis is crucial. Once you have got that you are halfway to getting things under control.

Types of lupus

Lupus is a condition that is known as the great mimic because it can appear to be lots of other diseases (*see also pages 28 and 53*). It is often mistaken for rheumatoid arthritis or multiple sclerosis, for instance. It can take time and a great deal of expertise to get a conclusive diagnosis. You have to add into that equation the fact that within lupus itself there are a number of different manifestations of the disease, some more severe than others. Once again there are no answers as to why one person with lupus should just have skin problems while another develops kidney disease. To complicate things further still it is possible for the different types of lupus to overlap, so you might have been diagnosed with discoid lupus that only affects the skin, but on top of that go on to develop SLE, which attacks internal tissue and organs.

Systemic lupus erythematosus (SLE, or LE)

This is the 'big brother' of the various lupuses because it is the most serious, working on the inner parts of the body, in particular major organs and body tissue. Here it will be referred to as lupus, or SLE. In its most dangerous form it can be a killer, but it can alternatively be so mild as to be hardly noticeable. Most people affected by it fall in between these extremes. Improved diagnostic techniques and an increasingly refined use of drug treatments mean that the outlook for the vast majority of people with SLE is good. If you read medical documents on SLE some talk about patients being 'fortunate as these days they can expect to live for ten years or more'. That hardly sounds fortunate if you are only in your twenties, but don't despair. It is academic medical shorthand for saying that most people who have the condition can look forward to living a relatively normal life span.

There is currently no known cure for SLE, but there are numerous research projects under way across the world to find some answers. SLE can go into remission, although, as with so many things to do with lupus, no one is sure why this happens. Full remission, where the disease disappears altogether, is relatively rare. What is seen more often is partial remission, where disease activity stops and then reappears. It can be that the affected person has numerous flares over a period of twelve months and then nothing for years.

There is one area where there is some evidence for why the disease might peter out, which is seen in post-menopausal women. There appears to be a link between the active disease and the female hormone oestrogen (*see page 20*), and it is quite common to see SLE calm down in women once they have been through the menopause and are producing less of this hormone. They can go on to develop the non-life-threatening discoid lupus (*see page 10*), or go into total remission and have no further problems. To date this aspect of lupus has come to light due to clinical observation, in other words as patients have got older doctors have witnessed the disease either weakening or stopping its activity. As yet there has not been formal research into why this happens.

Years ago SLE was considered a 'big name, small print' disease by the medical profession – in other words uncommon and not to be bothered with. These days the frequency of the condition is becoming more and more clear as there is increasing awareness of lupus globally. Improved diagnostic tests have also revealed that lupus is widespread. One of the most shocking facts that is often quoted among doctors in this field is that lupus is more common than leukaemia, HIV and multiple sclerosis (MS) *put together*. This is hard to believe when you consider that lupus is by far the least known of these conditions – there is still a long way to go before doctors consider lupus as a possible diagnosis in the first instance.

The 'systemic' part of the disorder's name means 'all over the body'; it is generalised and not specific to any one area. 'Erythema' means a redness of the skin. The word 'lupus' means wolf in Latin – it is thought that the name was first used in the nineteenth century, either because the facial rash made a sufferer look wolf-like, or because of the lesions on the skin that resembled the bite of an animal. Another common visual feature of lupus is what doctors call a 'butterfly rash' that spreads across the cheeks and the bridge of the nose – this is regarded as one of the classic signs that the disease is present in a patient.

SLE can affect the whole body, both inside and out. It can be very mild, causing symptoms like joint pain and a variety of rashes, such as itchy raised patches on the skin, or it can attack major organs, in particular the kidneys, heart, lungs and/or brain. What can be particularly frustrating is how the condition can come and go without warning. Those affected can have one flare and then nothing for years, or they can suffer repeated flares over a period of months. The symptoms can also change with each attack and they can be so widespread across the body that sufferers can feel overwhelmed by the number of things wrong with them. Lupus can be a 'top-to-toe' condition so it is important to know what to look out for (*see page 31* for a more detailed description of the symptoms).

Discoid lupus erythematosus (DLE)

DLE is sometimes referred to as 'cutaneous lupus'. It is the not-so-pretty face of lupus, causing a particular type of rash that can leave permanent scarring. It is a distressing condition because the angry red markings it makes are noticeable and are often on parts of the skin that are visible. Sometimes you see patients in lupus clinic waiting areas who have covered their faces because they feel so embarrassed about the state of their skins. Sufferers can become reclusive, refusing to leave their homes because of how they look.

Discoid means 'disc-like', and refers to the circular markings on the skin that thicken and later scar. They usually appear on exposed areas of skin like the face, neck and arms. They are also found on the fingers and feet, where the skin can become so thin that it cracks and is sore. The rash may occur in areas of the body that are usually covered, like the back and chest, as well as behind the ears or on the scalp. DLE can lead to hair loss and permanent bald patches. Nasty as it is, the thing to remember with DLE is that, unlike SLE, it is not life threatening. The discoid lesions are also a feature of SLE; the difference here is that the skin will usually clear up with appropriate treatment with out leaving scars.

It is estimated that between 5 and 10 per cent of DLE cases also have SLE and that the same percentage will go on to develop SLE. No one knows why this is the case and to date there is no way of guessing who will be affected; nor is there any way of preventing this from happening. What can be done is to look out for any major changes in the pattern of the disease. Both sufferers and doctors need to monitor the DLE closely to catch any progression towards SLE early on. It has also been observed in lupus clinics that where SLE has gone into remission in later life the person can go on to develop DLE.

A variety of rashes is a feature of lupus in general, so blood tests, skin biopsies and clinical observation by a doctor are required to establish which type a patient has.

Drug-induced lupus

Drug-induced lupus is rare and can be tricky to spot as it can closely mimic SLE. The list of prescription drugs that are implicated in triggering drug-induced lupus is a long one. When seeing your specialist it is crucial that you know the names of all the medications you have been taking so that they can check if there is a possible link. Having said that, do not be tempted to stop medication without first talking to your doctor; this is a highly specialised area and guesswork can be dangerous. The drugs that are known to cause this type of lupus include:

- **Hydralazine** An antihypertensive drug used to treat high blood pressure.
- **Procainamide** An antiarrhythmic drug that is used to regulate heart rhythm in tachycardia (abnormally rapid heartbeat).
- **Sulphasalazine** Used in colitis, Crohn's disease and rheumatoid arthritis.
- **Minocycline** A tetracycline antibiotic drug used to treat acne.

SLE symptoms will often appear after a person has been on high doses of these medications for some time, usually a number of years. They can experience fever, joint pain, skin rashes and fatigue, although they are unlikely to have any major organ involvement. There are a number of ways of establishing whether the condition is drug-induced lupus, the main one being through blood tests. The results will be different from those found in true lupus. Another method that doctors use of establishing that a patient has drug-induced lupus is to stop the medication they suspect is causing the problems. If the medication is the guilty party the symptoms disappear quite quickly – over a period of weeks or months.

There is a second type of drug-induced lupus that is once again extremely rare but is not so easily reversed. This is where certain medications can exacerbate underlying true lupus. In other words, you have the disease but it is dormant, possibly undiagnosed, and a drug can kick-start a flare. In this case the drug will trigger an autoimmune reaction and once the lupus is active there is no way of turning the clock back – all that can be done is to treat it. Certain antibiotics can produce this effect, particularly Septrin, which is an antibacterial drug used to treat infections of the urinary and respiratory tracts, as well as of the gut, skin and ears.

If you know you have lupus you should be very careful about what medications you take. If you suspect you might have lupus and have 'classic' symptoms without a diagnosis and are on any of the above medications – or on any antibiotic – it is worth mentioning this to your doctor.

Neo-natal lupus

This is the rarest form of lupus, and although it can be frightening for new parents it is the least worrying. The neo-natal period is the first month of a baby's life. In that time an infant can develop a mild, lupus-like rash. What has happened is that an antibody – a protein made by white blood cells to fight alien microorganisms – in the mother's blood has passed to the baby via the placenta. This has triggered a reaction in the infant and led to the rash. Neo-natal lupus clears by the time an affected baby is about eight months old as the antibody causing the rash will have passed out of the baby's system. There is no evidence that this condition means the child will have lupus in later years. There are more details about lupus and pregnancy in Chapter 9 (*see page 131*).

Late-onset lupus

Although the majority of lupus cases occur in women of child-bearing age the disease can make an appearance in people of any age. When lupus occurs in people over the age of fifty-five, it is called late-onset lupus. It accounts for roughly 15 per cent of people with SLE. It is likely that a number of those who first show signs of lupus at over fifty years of age have had the disease for years before this but that it has been undetected. Late-onset lupus generally occurs in people of fifty-five upwards, and the disease is generally milder than the earlier form, with symptoms that are similar to those listed above but less severe. Correspondingly, the medications used are milder so there are fewer side effects. One problem is that lupus at this stage in life can be even harder to diagnose than at an earlier stage, as it mimics other diseases that are common in older age, like rheumatoid arthritis. Also, drug-induced lupus is more common in older people than in younger ones as they take more medications for high blood pressure and heart disease.

Who gets it?

Lupus is a common disease. In Britain it is estimated that there are currently 50,000 cases but that figure is increasing all the time due to growing awareness and better diagnostic techniques. Experts think that the number could easily be double this estimate. In the US the official figures indicate that more than a million people have lupus, but the key charities believe that the real number is closer to two million.

Lupus can affect men and women of any age. It can sometimes be seen in infants and appears in people aged over sixty, but the majority of cases are found in young people, in particular young women. Nine out of ten sufferers are female, with the highest incidence occurring between the ages of fifteen and forty-five. According to the charity Lupus UK, there is one case per 700 among women in general, but for high-risk groups that figure is one in 250. The ratio between the sexes alters outside the child-bearing years. It is more like three girls to one boy in children under twelve. This reflects the activity of the female hormone oestrogen, which is much more active in women post-puberty and pre-menopause.

Those considered to be at the highest risk are women of child-bearing age, post-puberty and pre-menopause. Within that group those who are particularly prone to lupus are women of Afro-Caribbean or Asian origin (*see pages 158*). Dr Hughes says that lupus is as much a black person's disease as sickle cell anaemia – in fact, lupus is more common but less recognised.

No one knows why certain ethnic groups are more prone to lupus than others, or why the disease is becoming more prevalent, but once again it could have a lot to do with the environment we have developed for ourselves. One interesting theory is that as we live cleaner lives our immune systems may be inexperienced. For instance, the reason lupus is less common in Africa than in the West is that children there have been exposed to lots of bugs. Their environment is loaded with different infectious elements and the majority of children will have come across a broad spectrum of germs from day one of their lives. They will therefore have developed a pretty tough immunity. In the West, on the other hand, every effort is made to kill as many bugs as possible, especially around babies. The knock-on effect of this is that the immune system doesn't get experience, so it isn't used to dealing with such a great spectrum of bugs. We are immunised and protected from infection, and the impact of this is that our inexperienced immune systems can become dysfunctional. Essentially, it means we are too clean!

★ ★ ★

Having established what the main types of lupus are and who is most at risk of getting it, we now move on to the subject of possible reasons why the condition occurs in some people, and what can trigger a flare.

Chapter 2

The Triggers

The cause of lupus is not known despite extensive ongoing research. No one is absolutely certain why one person gets it and not their neighbour. There are lots of theories and when you ask your doctor what has caused your lupus the reply is likely to be that it has something to do with genetics, the environment, a viral trigger or all three. It is believed that a person can inherit a predisposition to lupus – that it can be built into their DNA and make them likely to develop this autoimmune disease. You do see it running in families, in particular down the female line. It is more than chance that there are families with a mother and daughter or two sisters who have lupus. We know there is an increased incidence in identical twins. We have established that there is a lupus gene, or genes; they are complex, but are being mapped out quite closely now.

It is estimated that the chances of relatives of people with lupus developing the disease are anything between 5 and 10 per cent. This doesn't mean your daughter or granddaughter will necessarily develop it, but it is worth keeping an eye out for the telltale symptoms. A study carried out in the US with identical twins showed that where one had SLE the other had a 25 per cent chance of also having it or going on to develop it. The conclusion drawn from this was that it confirmed that lupus runs in families, but that there must be other factors involved – if the link was only down to genes then both twins would either have or not have SLE.

This reflects how complex the whole genetics question is. For instance, it is thought that we are dealing with not just one gene but a parcel of them – so it could be that someone needs to have these multiple genes before they are susceptible to developing lupus. If we knew what the genes were we could pinpoint a cause of the disease. One positive thing that comes out of this knowledge is that a person who suspects they have lupus can check their family history – in particular their close female relatives. It could be that the clues you need to help get a diagnosis are within your family group.

What triggers a flare?

When doctors talk about a 'flare' they are referring to the disease being active, that is the symptoms of lupus are present and they can be mild or severe. In lupus you can have a major flare and then nothing for a long period of time, or you can have a series of flares one after the other. Lupus affects everyone differently, and each person who has the condition has their own particular profile of symptoms. You therefore have to work out which of the following could lead to a flare in your particular case.

If you can keep a record of the days and weeks leading up to the onset of an attack you might be able to isolate what has caused it, or has contributed to causing it. As lupus is incurable you have to deal with it as being a part of you, something that you monitor and learn to control.

Perhaps one of the most important things to take on board is that you are your own best doctor. You have the most at stake and know your body better than anyone else. If you know there is something specific that sparks symptoms you should be able to avoid it in future, whether it is a type of environment, a lifestyle, a kind of food or certain medications.

Sunlight

Traditionally, ultraviolet (UV) rays have been regarded as one of the most common triggers of lupus. It is important to stress how common this sensitivity is – estimates are that roughly 50 per cent of people who have lupus react to UV rays. As lupus symptoms can change, a person might have an adverse reaction to the sun on one occasion and not on another.

If you have lupus you need to exercise caution if you are going to sunbathe. The link with lupus and UV to some extent explains why skin problems with the condition are often found on the parts of the body that are exposed to the sun's rays – like the face, neck, hands, arms and legs. If this is a trigger for you there are obvious steps you can take to protect yourself; for instance, you can use a high-factor sun lotion or make-up that has a good sun filter in it. If you have had or are having a flare, even a mild one, you should resist the temptation to sunbathe – a few hours in the sun might give you the beginnings of a healthy-looking tan, but it could also be enough to exacerbate the condition.

This photosensitivity means that people who have lupus are also more likely to suffer from sunburn. Scientists know that the UV rays from the sun increase immune system response, so in a person with lupus that reaction will be amplified as the immune system is already overactive. Then again, people with lupus should not feel that they are consigned to a lifetime in the shadows covered up from head to toe in clothing. As with so many things in lupus, the condition can change. It might be that you are highly sun sensitive during a flare but not so much while in periods of remission. It is up to you to test how you are after a short time in the sun. If you feel the early signs of a flare, take cover; if not, just be cautious. Even if, as a lupus sufferer, you haven't had problems with the sun in the past, it is a good idea to be careful with the sun, and you should certainly avoid sunbeds.

Cheryl Marcus, the founder of Lupus UK, knows only too well how the sun can trigger a flare. More than thirty years ago she and her new husband, Martin, headed off to sunny Portugal for their honeymoon. Within hours of hitting the sunbeds around the pool Cheryl was racked with pain as her joints became swollen and her skin inflamed. She spent most of her honeymoon lying in a cold bath – the only way she could get some relief from the pain. Her sensitivity to UV light, and being unaware that she had lupus, almost killed her.

Sex hormones

Hormones are now known to have a key influence on lupus, although no one knows exactly why. Once again a lot of research is under way into why the female hormone oestrogen and its male counterpart testosterone are linked so closely with the immune system. Laboratories across the world are looking at this question using selected breeds of mice that have lupus (certain mammals are prone to the disease, including dogs, mice, monkeys and horses). When the mice are given oestrogen their condition worsens, while with testosterone they improve. That sounds fairly simplistic, but there is nothing simple about this disease.

The research is not something that could be applied to humans at this stage, but it is an important confirmation that sex hormones hold essential clues to what triggers lupus and why it affects so many more women than men. Women are tuned in to their menstrual cycles, and lupus sufferers often feel worse towards the end of a cycle, when their oestrogen levels are high. If the lupus begins to grumble – for instance if you begin to feel abnormally fatigued and your joints are sore – it is a warning that a flare might be imminent.

Another dangerous time for women is after childbirth. It is estimated that as many as 25 per cent of cases first appear in a woman just after giving birth, a time which doctors call the puerperium. It is thought that this is due to the increased hormonal activity during childbirth. There is, however, no formal scientific research – this is a view based on the high incidence of flares during this period. This is a particularly harsh aspect of lupus – it seems very cruel that a new mother may become so ill that she cannot enjoy her baby, and in some cases might be too unwell to even care for her child. The questions of hormones, pregnancy and lupus are dealt with in Chapter 9, which looks at women and lupus in more depth.

Stress

When you speak to people with lupus they invariably feel that the disease appeared during or shortly after a period of extreme stress. Not so long ago the suggestion that bereavement might have made you actually physically sick would have been 'pooh poohed' by doctors, but that is changing. The team at St Thomas' Hospital lupus clinic have no doubt that stress is a crucial factor in triggering a flare. They have noted that many patients can pinpoint their worsening health to a particular occasion or event in their lives. Patients turn up who have suffered a terrible flare after a bereavement or a major upset like losing their job. Time and again when someone recounts how their health has worsened they will link it to an actual event.

The close link between brain and body function is now well recognised, and research supports the view that your state of mind and the way your immune system works are tied in. Stress can have an impact on heart rate, breathing, blood pressure and energy levels.

Of course, telling people to avoid stress is a bit like asking someone to bow out of contemporary life; it isn't possible or feasible. Facing bereavement, job loss or major upheavals are part and parcel of most people's existence. A person with lupus can, however, try and limit exposure to activities or situations that they find stressful. For instance, if your job is highly pressurised explore ways of making it less so – if you work a tough shift pattern see if you can change it. You could look for another job. This may be easier said than done, but it might be what you need to do to control the lupus better. At a time of particular stress look out for the early signs of a flare and cater for them.

Angie Davidson was immersed in managing a pub when she first became seriously ill ten years ago. With her then husband she was working long hours, and even when she was resting the stresses of running a business never left her. Angie – who is now the campaign director of St Thomas' Lupus Trust – can pinpoint the start of her first major lupus flare to a particular morning back in 1993, although it was to be years before she could put a name to what was wrong with her. Angie has no doubt that severe stress is what triggered her lupus.

On this particular morning I woke up feeling that I had the world's worst case of flu. I had always been very healthy in my life. I certainly had never been in hospital and never complained when I had minor ailments, so the fact that I insisted on seeing a doctor is a clue to how ill I was. I was frustrated that the GP didn't examine me; she just recommended rest and aspirin or something similar. I went home but was no better; I felt as though I had gone ten rounds with Frank Bruno and lost the lot. I had been working incredibly hard at the time. I was running a pub so the hours were long and pressurised. I never took time off, and being unwell was just not an option. I know I was highly stressed but I didn't connect the way I was feeling with anything more serious — not at first anyway.

Angie was finally diagnosed with lupus four years later (see pages 26–8).

Drugs and chemicals

For many years there has been debate in the UK and the US about whether certain chemicals found in commonly used products can act as lupus triggers. For instance, there has been research into links with lipstick, food colouring, hair dyes and tobacco smoke. To date there is nothing that supports a connection, although the nature of lupus is that it makes a person highly 'allergic'. This might make them more likely to react to substances like colouring in products. Once again it is important for the person with lupus to track what scientists call 'cause and effect', in other words what you ate or were exposed to in the run-up to a flare, and make sure you avoid it in future.

As described in Chapter 1 (*see page 12*), certain medications can trigger lupus or symptoms that appear to be lupus.

This is extremely rare but if you are taking certain drugs, in particular antibiotics, it is worth checking for a possible connection.

Viruses and bacteria

There is a lot of research under way into the question of whether lupus is triggered by a virus or bacteria. Dr Bob Lahita, from New Jersey City Medical Center in the US, ranks alongside Dr Hughes of London's St Thomas' Hospital as one of the world's leading experts in this condition. Dr Lahita has spent years looking into the question of a viral or bacterial trigger. He is convinced that the disease is 'infectious' – not in the sense that you catch it, but that some people are predisposed to lupus. So if a foreign agent – such as a virus or bacteria – enters the body of someone who is susceptible to lupus, their immune system can react abnormally and thereby trigger the disease, making it active.

If Dr Lahita is right then tracking down the infectious particle – or particles – that cause lupus could lead not only to better treatment but also to something even more desirable – a cure. It would also be a breakthrough for other autoimmune conditions. Finding out what causes SLE is the essential first step towards discovering how to switch off the destructive overactive immune system. At the moment all doctors can do is treat the symptoms.

To date the idea of the infectious nature of lupus is a theory formulated by leading doctors after years of hands-on experience with patients. Despite extensive studies, there is no published research available yet to bear out this theory or indicate what the infectious trigger is, although it certainly seems possible that this line of research could come up with some badly needed answers.

★　★　★

The next chapter tackles the complex subject of the many symptoms of lupus and the current difficulties in obtaining a diagnosis.

Chapter 3

Lupus Symptoms

Getting a diagnosis is the 'Holy Grail' of the lupus world. Without it you find yourself bounced from one specialist to another, often clutching a fistful of painkillers and antidepressants. In the years since my diagnosis I have spoken to hundreds of people with lupus and almost every single one has had a nightmare finding out what was wrong with them. In some cases it has taken decades for the doctors to come to the conclusion that lupus was behind the myriad painful symptoms; for others the diagnosis remains frustratingly illusive.

Here is how Angie Davidson, who has already been mentioned in Chapter 2, experienced her symptoms before she was finally diagnosed:

> [For many years] I never really felt completely well. It was hard to say why and sometimes I couldn't really put my finger on what exactly it was. I certainly felt depressed, which was weird, as I was usually very upbeat. I was also constantly exhausted. When I say that, I don't mean like after a late night. I was exhausted and could sleep and sleep as many hours as I was allowed. I was annoyed with myself as I thought I was being lazy. I had attacks of what I could only describe as

'flu-like' symptoms, where I just felt generally very ill. I also began to get night sweats and regular migraines. I then developed aches similar to 'growing pains'. I couldn't seem to sit comfortably at all and I'd spend all night fidgeting.

During this time I developed what I thought was a severe toothache. I went to the dentist who said I needed root canal work. A few weeks after the treatment I returned saying the pain was back as bad as ever. The dentist said I had no nerves under the tooth and it was impossible. I assured him the pain was real. Yet another 'medical professional' whom I couldn't convince I had a problem! I was then sent to a specialist in Harley Street who also could find nothing. Overall the treatment cost over £500, and not once did any of the dentists suggest I consult a doctor to see what was causing the pain.

I finally developed severe pains in my knees and then in my hands, to the extent where I couldn't hold anything that weighed more than a few ounces, as it was too painful.

During this whole period I had been visiting the doctor on a regular basis (weekly or monthly). It was annoying as I couldn't seem to convince him that something was wrong, although in my heart I knew I had a problem. Also, typical of lupus patients, I looked really well.

I didn't know it but I was showing all the classic symptoms of lupus: mouth ulcers, depression, exhaustion, joint/muscle pains, night sweats and migraines. The usual misdiagnosis in the case of female lupus sufferers is that they are having hormone problems; change of life, etc. I was convinced this was not what was wrong with me, but no one had any answers and they didn't believe that I had a serious health problem. Many lupus sufferers are treated as hypochondriacs or (as I was) offered 'counselling' – which I took to mean that they thought I was crazy. Finally, when I had very severe pains in my hands, which then moved into my knee joints, the doctor referred me to an arthritis clinic.

It was at this stage that I was lucky enough to be seen by Dr David D'Cruz, a rheumatologist who is also a lupus specialist. To my sheer relief he recognised the symptoms immediately. One simple positive blood test and I had the reason for all the problems! My feeling after being told I had lupus was one of relief. I was very close to actually believing that I was going insane and that the symptoms were all in my mind. Now I had a name for my illness and no matter how bad that was at least I knew what I was up against. From the point of the first big flare to getting a diagnosis had taken four years.

A multitude of symptoms

Lupus is the type of disease where you could read the list of symptoms below and think 'Yeah, that's me. I have some of those problems; that's what I have got,' but it isn't that simple. Lupus is a great mimic. It is often mistaken for multiple sclerosis (MS), rheumatoid arthritis or myalgic encephalomyelitis (ME). Of course, that can work both ways, so it is important to be cautious before a firm diagnosis is arrived at. For instance, there are a number of people – mostly women – who have been told that they have lupus when in fact they are suffering from fibromyalgia (*see page 60*). This is a worrying mistake as both diseases share symptoms, but the degree of severity and treatment are quite different.

The only thing worse than not getting a diagnosis is being wrongly diagnosed. It is important that people are not put in a convenient 'autoimmune slot'. By that I mean being told they have lupus because their disparate array of symptoms fits the bill and not because an expert in the field has reached that conclusion. On the flip side the difficulty of spotting lupus and the limited awareness of it can result in it being overlooked or rejected as a diagnosis.

These days you can get your hands on a phenomenal amount of information via the Internet, but don't be tempted to diagnose yourself and thereby become convinced you have a certain condition. Lupus is a tricky disease to spot even for the medical experts, so a layperson will certainly struggle. The key is to get some balance; doctors and patients must work together. With so many issues at stake it is essential that the right tests are carried out and that the patient sees someone who is a specialist in this field. In the UK you'll need to see a rheumatology specialist because this is the speciality that has traditionally dealt with lupus.

There are several conditions that fall under the auto-immune umbrella, covering all areas of the health spectrum (these are looked at more fully in Chapter 4). You will find that your doctors are quite rightly careful about handing out a diagnosis of SLE without having the back-up of clinical and physiological tests – in particular blood tests. There are few, if any, cases where a doctor will take one look at a patient and say, 'This is a classic case of lupus, my dear – here, take these steroids and give me a call in the morning.' It just doesn't happen that way, even when someone has the most recognised symptom of lupus – the butterfly rash across their cheeks and the bridge of their nose. Other diseases can cause a facial rash.

To reach the conclusion that it is lupus a doctor has to take an overall view of each case. As a patient you need to know that getting a diagnosis is a process of elimination. When endless tests come back negative it can be disheartening, not because you want them to be positive but because the questions remain unanswered and you still feel unwell. The tests are not a pointless exercise – all those results are crucial as they help cross things off the list. As your doctor searches for the answers you can assist by preparing well for appointments. You will have waited many months to see a specialist who is pressed for time, so make the most of it. The action plan (*see page 177*) provides advice from consultants on how you can help them help you.

It is possible – indeed likely – that you will have to fight to get a name for your condition. When I interview female lupus sufferers they frequently mention how they have been fobbed off by their doctor, and that they believe they have not been taken seriously. This could have a lot to do with the fact that most of those who have lupus are women and that the first presenting symptoms are often chronic fatigue and depression, both of which are invisible and hard to pinpoint.

A diagnostic puzzle

Lupus has many faces; it can attack a number of different areas of the body at one time, and in each flare the symptoms can vary. Hence people who have lupus can have many things wrong with them. People often tell me how they were so embarrassed about the number and variety of their ailments that they even began to doubt themselves and wondered if they were imagining things.

If you put all these factors together you can see why lupus is such a tricky disease to pin down. The odds are stacked against someone getting a speedy diagnosis. The hurdles are: widespread ignorance and the complexity of the condition.

Top to toe – the symptoms of lupus

To the uninitiated the number of symptoms in SLE can read a bit like a medical dictionary as potentially every part of the body can be affected. Patients can find themselves seeing a bewildering variety of different specialists, from neurologists to cardiologists. One male lupus sufferer joked to me that he had seen every kind of 'ologist' with the exception of a gynaecologist. The best way of ensuring that your case is dealt with efficiently is for it to come under one leading physician. In the case of lupus this will usually be a consultant rheumatologist. That way the results of various tests and consultations will find their way back to the one department and they can be used in conjunction with other investigations and treatments. If you feel you are being passed from one specialist to another and they are not coordinating with each other, you should discuss your concerns with your doctor.

Main symptoms

- chronic fatigue,
- joint pain or swelling,
- skin rashes,
- fever,
- major organ involvement – kidney, brain/ CNS, heart,
- neurological problems,
- ulcers,
- depression,
- headaches,
- UVA sensitivity,
- blood abnormalities.

Chronic fatigue or malaise

This is one of the most common and debilitating lupus symptoms, and sadly the one that is often overlooked. It is

31

hard to describe what utter exhaustion feels like, but if you have experienced it you will know how devastating it can be. You wake in the morning feeling as though you are glued to your bed, unable to get up. Your brain is ticking away but your body does not respond to the call to action. There are times when you struggle to get up a flight of stairs, wrestling for breath as though you have just run a marathon. Simple daily tasks become chores beyond your wildest dreams. Life slips by and you are too weak to grasp your share of it. Worse still is the fact that those around you cannot understand how tired you are – exhaustion isn't something you can see.

A new study carried out by the Rayne Institute at St Thomas' Hospital has looked at fatigue. The findings showed that the best way to combat this symptom was to do exercise. In the past doctors advised people to have long periods of bed rest. The study is now making them rethink that guidance. It obviously depends on how active the lupus is – for example, someone with badly inflamed joints and a fever would not be able to do exercise. For someone who is reasonably mobile, however, the advice goes something like 'On your bike or take a hike.'

What emerged from the above study was that the main factor involved in fatigue in relation to lupus was disease activity, so that the more active the disease is, the more likely you are to feel fatigued. This would seem obvious, but it is not clear in the current literature; there are some studies that claim that fatigue has nothing to do with disease activity. However, 95 per cent of patients in the study had significant fatigue – not just a bit of tiredness at the end of the day, but pathological fatigue. By this I mean a physical feeling of fatigue involving the inability to get on and do things, rather than merely a lack of motivation. Another significant driver of fatigue is depression and 30 per cent of lupus sufferers will have depression at any one time. Abnormal sleep patterns also contribute to fatigue, and over 50 per cent of people with lupus have trouble with sleep.

Metabolic problems – thyroid disorders, for instance – are common in lupus sufferers. Both an underactive and an overactive thyroid can give you fatigue, as can anaemia, which is seen in 20 per cent of people with lupus. Finally, in a large portion of cases, it is not known what causes it.

Consultant rheumatologist Dr David D'Cruz was involved in the study and he feels that in the light of the results doctors will have to look again at the advice they give to patients in relation to taking exercise. To quote Dr D'Cruz:

The study found that in general terms lupus patients were very unfit. This could be because they have got into a vicious cycle because they are tired and unwell so they don't exercise. The other part of the explanation could be that we have been at fault in the past by telling patients who are feeling tired and unwell to go to bed and rest. This study reveals that it may be wrong to give such general advice, which in the end could prove to be counterproductive.

We examined this question by doing a randomised study looking at three groups of patients. Some we did nothing with; another group were given an exercise routine monitored by Dr Colin Tench, who ran the trial. A third group was asked to relax with relaxation tapes – they came to classes and did stretches but nothing more vigorous. The results were quite clear. The ones who exercised reported an improvement in their general condition in relation to fatigue. More than 50 per cent said they felt 'better' or 'very much better' with an exercise programme.

Painful or swollen joints and muscle pain

Next to fatigue, aching joints is one of the most important symptoms of lupus, seen in more than 90 per cent
of lupus sufferers. It is also quite common for people who
become ill with lupus in their twenties or thirties to have
had sore joints when they were much younger, although
this would generally have been put down to 'growing
pains'. Joint pain is like an early warning that lupus is
becoming active. It is often the case that a person has
suffered varying degrees of discomfort in the major and
minor joints for months or years before other symptoms
appear. Any of the joints can be affected, the most common
being the knees, hips, shoulders, elbows, fingers and toes.
In people with lupus you often see puffy fingers, toes and
knees.

You will hear the term 'lupus arthritis' used by doctors.
Arthritis means inflammation of the joints and there are different types of arthritis. In lupus, unlike in rheumatoid arthritis (*see page 62*), this inflammation does not usually lead to
permanent damage to bone and cartilage. Lupus arthritis
causes temporary swelling that is generally reversible. With
treatment, the cartilage usually reverts to its normal size. It
is seen in almost 50 per cent of people with lupus. The stiffness is more pronounced at either end of the day, and is
usually symmetrical – affecting the same joints on both sides
of the body. If someone has just one joint that is swollen
and painful, this is unlikely to be caused by the lupus.

On rare occasions inflammation of the tendons in the
finger joints can lead to some long-term deformity. Tendon
stiffness can be a recurring problem, affecting activities such
as typing, piano playing and so on. It is these hand joints
that can be most noticeably disfigured – there is a classic
lupus condition called 'hitchhiker's thumb' where both

thumbs bend over backwards. It looks nasty, but medication will bring down the swelling.

The pain often comes and goes. Some people say it is worse in cold weather, but there is no strong evidence to support the claim that climate influences this form of arthritis. In fact, although the sun is a trigger for lupus it can be that the joint pains actually feel better in the warmth.

Rashes or odd skin colouration

Rashes are the 'hallmark' of lupus. As mentioned previously, one of the classic indicators that lupus might be present is the butterfly rash that covers the cheeks and the bridge of the nose. About 80 per cent of people with lupus have some kind of cutaneous or skin involvement. In lupus there are several different types of rash. At the milder end of the spectrum are itchy hives, which usually appear on the tips of the fingers and toes. At the other end is discoid lupus, where round, coin-like lesions develop that can become hard and leave scars. The rashes in SLE can be similar; the difference is that is they usually disappear once a flare is under control.

There is one other skin change that is significant in lupus, called livedo reticularis. This is a marbling of the skin, which occurs as red and white blotches that appear in a lace-like pattern, usually on the wrists and knees. This skin condition is found in about 20 per cent of cases. Doctors look for livedo reticularis because it shows that the blood vessels near the skin have been affected. It is seen most frequently in people who also have Hughes syndrome, or sticky blood (*see page 54*).

Vasculitis (inflamed blood vessels)

It is common in lupus for the small blood vessels to become inflamed – as with livedo reticularis it is possible to recognise disease activity through the skin colouration. Cutaneous vasculitis is the inflammation of the superficial blood vessels near the skin. This is one of the main features of lupus, seen in up to 70 per cent of people who have the condition. Doctors refer to it as 'vasculitis'. It can be observed where blood vessels are affected in the fingertips and elbows, and around the eyes.

Vasculitis can manifest itself as painful black spots on the fingertips, blood spots on the legs and ulcers on the lower limbs. You can also get painful black spots on the earlobes, the backs of the elbows and the feet. These are the classic places where vasculitis can appear. The black spots are areas of skin that is actually dead – they occur because the inflammation narrows the blood vessels and thereby cuts off the blood supply, causing the areas of skin to die.

Usually the lesions heal over completely once the disease is treated. However, they are an indicator that something very serious is going on.

Some people find that the whites of their eyes – known as the sclera – go red because the fine blood vessels to the eyes have become inflamed. This is a rare condition known as scleritis, which needs to be dealt with quickly to avoid any permanent damage to the eyes.

Fever

The normal body temperature of a healthy, resting adult is 98.6 degrees Fahrenheit, or 37.0 degrees Celsius. Although the body temperature can vary slightly on an individual basis, the range is limited. In people with lupus it is common to find that when having a flare they have a low-grade fever, during which their body temperature is raised by one or two degrees. Depending on the person, this can cause discomfort or go relatively unnoticed. Some people suffer from night sweats, even when their body temperature is relatively normal. These symptoms are an indicator that the disease is likely to be active. In women with lupus a slight fever or raised temperature in the run-up to a period is not uncommon and could be the cause of night sweats.

Effects on the central nervous system (CNS)

Up until thirty years ago it was thought that the brain was not affected by lupus. The medical wisdom was that this vital but delicate organ was protected by the 'blood brain barrier' (BBB), and that this kept out 'hooligan' autoimmune cells that did so much damage to other parts of the body. Without going into a lot of technical detail, the opinion was that specialised blood vessels supplying the brain, which formed the BBB, prevented the brain from being affected by lupus.

This viewpoint could not have been more wrong. Since the early 1970s the impact of lupus on the brain has become widely recognized, to the extent that it is now thought that a staggering 90 per cent of people with lupus have some kind of neurological involvement. The central nervous system – often referred to as the CNS – includes both the brain and the spinal cord and is a common target of lupus. The involvement of the brain is sometimes called 'cerebral lupus'. The peripheral nervous system – which involves the skin and muscles – can also be affected. For instance, the hands, feet and parts of the face can become numb or so oversensitive that they cannot be touched.

Leading consultant neurologist Dr Mohammed Sharief works closely with the lupus clinic at St Thomas' Hospital.

In the past the brain was labelled as being an 'immunologically privileged site'; it was protected by the blood brain barrier so it was thought that it was well away from the hassle and dangers of lupus. It turns out that the immune privilege is a curse rather than an advantage because the brain has no local defence – if the lupus invades the brain then there is nothing to stop it causing damage. The brain is defenceless. . . . now we know that more than 90 per cent of people with lupus suffer from neurological symptoms and these can range from mild headaches, numbness and dizziness to major psychotic episodes.

Dr Sharief agrees that awareness is the key to diagnosing CNS lupus. He feels that his fellow neurologists need to consider lupus more often, especially when they see a patient who has a variety of unexplained symptoms.

I saw an elderly woman last year who came in with what I was told was CJD – the human form of mad cow disease. Her hands were trembling, her legs moving constantly, and she could not speak or control her own movements. Still I was not happy with this diagnosis so I did further tests and it transpired that in fact she had CNS lupus and Hughes syndrome. (See page 54.) Once she was treated the symptoms were brought under control.

Dr Sharief says he understands why so many people who eventually arrive at his door are bitter – a lot of them have been passed from department to department and made to feel that they are neurotic. He says a patient who suspects they have lupus should insist that the relevant blood tests are carried out to establish whether this disease is present and active. In his own surprisingly candid words, 'Doctors are there as servants to the patient.'

The neurological involvement is vast. By neuro I mean any symptom which may suggest brain involvement . . . I personally think that the majority of people who suffer from lupus will eventually have some neuro symptoms. These could be as mild as dizziness or headaches or as devastating as dementia or paralysis . . . What the symptoms are depends on the duration of the disease, the extent of treatment and the associated inflammation with lupus. So for example those patients who have antiphospholipid syndrome [explained in Chapter 4] as part of lupus will have more risk of neurological problems. In this I also include psychiatric or neuro psychiatric problems because I believe that there is a fine or hazy line between neurology and psychiatry. Psychiatric symptoms may be a manifestation of neurological disease and vice versa.

The most extreme but uncommon symptoms are multiple damage to the brain, which can cause strokes, dementia and blindness in lupus. Lupus may affect various parts of the brain individually and that is because it affects the blood supply to the brain and causes local inflammation or mini strokes – TIAs – and therefore you cannot fit it in a recognised syndrome. . . . [Lupus] can present in any way possible depending on which part of the brain is affected. It is a diagnostic puzzle. If you don't think of lupus then you won't find it. *It is a puzzle and you have to fit all the pieces together in order to reach the diagnosis.*

Neurologists are finding that the number of cases of mild lupus is growing. Many of these patients wouldn't have come to a neurologist in the past. They usually have vague symptoms like dizziness, headache, poor concentration and tiredness during the day, non-specific things that anyone can feel. If a neurologist isn't vigilant enough then they could dismiss them again as depressed, neurotic, overworked or stressed out, but if there are other telltale symptoms, like movement difficulties, memory or speech problems, numbness or odd behaviour, then you must check the blood; there is a chance you will find that lupus is what is causing all this.

39

To hear that your brain has been affected by a disease is frightening, and the key thing you want to know is whether the damage will be permanent. The answer is that this depends on what harm the disease has done. In lupus the damage can be due to inflammation or lack of blood supply. Problems that result from the latter or mini strokes are irreversible. The key in these cases is to prevent the spread of the disease and to encourage the remaining brain cells to take over. If, however, the damage is due to inflammation, then it is totally reversible. Medication to damp down the inflammation – like steroids – can reverse it 100 per cent.

Depression

The physical signs of depression are:

- Changes in appetite for life/food/sex.
- Problems in sleeping.
- Low mood, especially on waking.
- Inability to concentrate.
- Agitation.

Depression is common in lupus. It isn't always easy to know for sure whether it is part of the disease or part of your reaction to having the disease. Whichever way around, the symptoms end up in a relentless cycle that has to be broken. As in the case of any emotional rollercoaster, you have to deal with what is pressing the 'start' button and get it to 'stop'.

You might have already come across doctors who dismiss the depression on the basis that you are 'bound to feel blue when you have a condition like lupus'. That might well be the case, but if ignored this low mood can go on and develop into a serious reactive depression that must be treated. Persuading a doubting GP can be problematic and this might mean you don't get the help you want and need for depression. Knowing what to look for to spot genuine depression will help.

The physical signs of depression (summarised briefly above) include changes in your 'appetite' for life, food or sex. You could find that you have problems sleeping and that you wake up feeling depressed. You might be agitated or experience such a lack of concentration that you can't read a book or watch television. Those who have severe depression find that nothing will lift their mood; they feel despair and a sense of hopelessness, and can suffer from self-loathing. If you are sick in this way then you are likely to need anti-depressants.

If you don't have these biological symptoms it may be that you are simply unhappy and medication will be less effective. In both cases you will need some form of support. This can range from talking to other patients or charities and getting comfort from sharing your experiences of lupus, to undergoing a more formal programme of counselling or psychotherapy. Some lupus clinics do offer psychological and psychiatric help. If yours does not, you can ask for the name of someone it would recommend whom you could see privately. It is important to ensure that whoever you see is knowledgeable about lupus. It is also crucial that you realise that depression is a real part of lupus; it is not just indulging in feeling a 'bit blue', but a condition that you have to take seriously.

Effects on the kidneys

Of all the body's major organs the kidneys can suffer the most permanent damage as a result of lupus. They are very delicate organs that have limited ability to recover, so it is crucial to monitor closely any impact the disease might be having, particularly bearing in mind how common attacks on the kidney are in lupus. It is estimated that up to 50 per cent of people who have lupus will have some degree of kidney involvement, called lupus nephritis by doctors. The most worrying aspect of the kidneys being affected is that this is generally a silent attack. By that I mean you are unlikely to feel any discomfort or pain.

Lupus can affect the kidneys in two ways – by attacking the fine filtration system or by making the blood vessels to the organs inflamed. A kidney reacts to an attack in a number of ways. It can allow proteins to leak into the urine, or impurities like urea and creatinine, which it would normally filter out of the system, can remain in the blood and accumulate. This only happens in severe cases and the person affected feels generally unwell, with nausea and weight loss. It is also common for blood pressure to rise when the kidneys are under attack.

Numerous standard tests can be carried out to keep an eye on the kidneys. The one that a person with lupus will be most familiar with involves providing a urine sample that is then tested with a dipstick. This checks for proteins, blood and other abnormal changes in the urine. At St Thomas' Hospital lupus clinic, patients are taught how to do their own urine tests so that they can monitor any changes themselves. Another way of spotting possible kidney problems is to check for oedema – an abnormal accumulation of fluid in body tissue. Signs of this include swollen ankles, face, fingers and/or abdomen. You might also have a general feeling of being bloated. If your kidneys are involved you may also experience headaches, frothy urine and possibly having a bloody nose.

The key to protecting the kidneys is to spot any problems early. The most serious cases are seen among people who have had lupus for years without a diagnosis and therefore without treatment. Having said that it is rare for someone to need dialysis or a transplant as a result of lupus. Even patients with active kidney disease can recover enough to get off medication.

Effects on the heart and lungs

Lupus can attack the sensitive linings of the heart and lungs, and once again this is quite common, affecting up to 50 per cent of lupus sufferers. The pericardium is the lining of the heart, so if it becomes inflamed you have pericarditis. In the lungs the lining is called the pleura, hence the name pleurisy when that is affected. These are painful conditions and can be frightening, as they can cause sharp chest pain when you breathe in deeply. You may find that you have to fight for breath, especially if there is a build-up of fluid around the linings. Although these symptoms can be worrying they respond well to treatment and are not in themselves life threatening.

Costochondritis (chest pains)

You may hear your doctor talk about costochondritis if you are having chest pain. This is an inflammation of the tissue that joins your ribs together at the breastbone and sternum. It can be very painful, especially when you breathe. It hurts to touch your ribs and it can be uncomfortable even when you are lying down. Any chest pain is scary, because you can find yourself panicking that it has something to do with your heart. But this symptom alone has nothing to do with cardiac function. Costochondritis on its own does not unduly worry doctors, but it is an indication that other things are going on in the body, and it will go with treatment.

Headaches

This is a common symptom that is often overlooked. It can be the case that a person has had a history of severe headaches dating back to their teenage years without any further investigation into them. It may be that they were the only symptom at the time. It is not uncommon to have someone diagnosed with lupus and then confirm that they had repeated severe headaches when they were younger. The lupus headache can also make an appearance as a full-blown migraine. The person will have all the migraine-like symptoms, which range from flashing lights, nausea and vomiting, to not being able to cope with normal light and having to hide away in a darkened room. They can also have lesser but similar migraine symptoms.

The headaches can be linked with the cross-over disease Hughes syndrome (*see page 54*). When the blood is prone to clotting it can lead to severe headaches. Some people call it a 'mind fog', which is cleared up once they take anticoagulants that are designed to thin the blood. The treatments for lupus and Hughes syndrome are effective against headaches brought on by these conditions.

Mouth or nose ulcers

Ulcers are common in lupus, so you will find that one of the first questions a specialist might ask is whether or not you have had mouth ulcers. They can also occur in the nose. As with skin changes, the presence of ulcers in someone with lupus is seen as an indication that the disease is flaring. Treatment for the lupus should help to resolve the ulcers, which can be very painful and make eating and drinking difficult. There are a number of mouthwashes that can help, or creams that can numb ulcers for a short period of time.

If they are very bad a doctor might give you a steroid lozenge or paste. When the ulcers appear in the nose a steroidal nasal spray might be used alongside petroleum jelly.

Doctors do recommend that you keep an eye on your oral hygiene to limit bacteria. You could use a softer toothbrush to limit the pain while ensuring that your teeth are kept clean. Dental care in lupus is important as some of the medications prescribed can have an impact on your gums. This is especially true if you have the cross-over condition Sjogren's syndrome (*see page 58*), in which less saliva is produced than normal so that the teeth and gums are at risk.

Effects on the gut

To date there has been little research into how lupus can affect the gut. Specialist clinics do see cases where SLE appears to have caused problems in this area of the body. It is possible that the result is a form of irritable bowel syndrome (IBS). Symptoms include diarrhoea – opening your bowels three or four times a day – abdominal pain and a grumbling, gurgling tummy. This could be due to a number of factors, such as a negative reaction to certain foods (lupus can make people highly allergic) or an adverse reaction to some of the medication. It is also possible for lupus to affect the gut by attacking the lining, although this is thought to be a rare symptom. Research is under way to try and establish what role lupus has in damage to the gut.

Hair loss

Hair loss, or alopecia, is quite common in systemic and discoid lupus. About 50 per cent of lupus sufferers experience some degree of hair loss either in patches around the scalp or as a generalised thinning of the hair. It is possible for someone to lose all their body hair – this is known as alopecia totalis – but it is rare and the hair generally grows back of its own accord. Doctors don't know what causes hair loss but it can be due to some of the medications that a person is on – in particular chemotherapy agents and steroids. Stress can also lead to alopecia and it is possible that the disease itself causes the hair follicles to be attacked under the scalp. Most of this hair loss is reversible, especially where it is caused by medication.

Blood disorders

For some people a blood disorder is the first indication that they have the disease. The following are the blood disorders most commonly linked with lupus:

- Anaemia is common. The red blood cell count is down, and you can look pale and feel fatigued as a result.

- Thrombocytopenia is a lowering in the number of platelets in the blood. Platelets are tiny particles that are necessary to prevent excessive bleeding by making the blood clot. In lupus the number of platelets can fall dramatically, leading to bleeding just under the skin. The small, reddish brown marks that are generally the size of a pinhead are called purpura.

- Sticky blood or Hughes syndrome (*see page 54*) is found in a third of people with lupus. The blood becomes more viscous and is therefore more likely to clot. This can lead to a myriad of symptoms, from deep vein thrombosis to recurrent miscarriage and stroke.

Medical criteria for recognising lupus

Because lupus is so difficult to identify, the American College of Rheumatology (ACR) published a list of criteria for recognising lupus in 1971. This list has been updated a number of times as knowledge about lupus has progressed, with the last changes being made a few years ago. Many books say that in order to diagnose lupus a person has to meet four of the eleven ACR criteria, and doctors do use this as a guide for diagnosis. However, sticking religiously to this list can be limiting. It was not drawn up as a diagnostic tool, but created as a means of helping to classify lupus. Using the criteria alone for diagnosis would be too restrictive – specialists need to look beyond a rigid list of symptoms.

The ACR's criteria for SLE are as follows:

- Rash over the cheeks (malar rash).
- Red raised patches (discoid rash).
- Photosensitivity.
- Mouth ulcers.
- Non-erosive arthritis.
- Inflammation of the lining of the lungs or heart (serositis).
- Excessive protein or other abnormal elements in the urine.
- Seizures or psychosis in the absence of other known causal factors.
- Low white blood cell, lymphocyte or platelet count.
- Positive test for antinuclear antibodies (*see page 66*).
- Positive test for anti-dsDNA, anti-Sm or antiphospholipid antibodies (*see pages 66–9*), or false positive syphilis test.

St Thomas' criteria for recognising lupus

The team at St Thomas' Hospital felt that because the ACR list was so limiting it would be useful to come up with supplementary criteria that could also be taken into consideration when making a diagnosis. This list is broader and draws on clinical experience with patients. Taking a good patient history is crucial in ascertaining whether a person fulfills these criteria.

- *Teenage 'growing pains'* It is quite common for people with lupus to recall that they had growing pains in their teens.

- *Teenage migraine* Classifying a 'headache' is notoriously difficult, but if a person talks about having a history of migraine or a cluster headache in their teens or early adult years, this is significant in a lupus context. It could also indicate the presence of Hughes syndrome (*see page 54*), which makes the blood more likely to clot and causes headaches.

- *Glandular fever* Prolonged glandular fever is a label that crops up time and time again in people with lupus and it is common to find that as children they will have had prolonged periods off school due to what was diagnosed as glandular fever but was in fact early lupus.

- *Severe reactions* to insect bites The clinic at St Thomas' sees a large number of patients who have a dramatic reaction to insect bites. As the skin is a major organ affected by lupus this isn't a surprising feature. It is, however, often overlooked because this kind of reaction is frequently also found in people without lupus.

- **Recurrent miscarriage** A third of lupus patients also have Hughes syndrome. One of the most prominent features of Hughes syndrome is multiple miscarriage. If a woman has suffered this kind of loss it is a strong indicator that she could have this condition and should also be tested for lupus.

- **Allergy to certain drugs** It is important to establish whether a person has had any adverse reaction to medications – like rashes, nausea or headaches in particular when taking the antibacterial drugs that contain sulphonamide or Septrin, which are used for urinary tract infections.

- **Agoraphobia/claustrophobia** Neurological problems are common in lupus. Sufferers often give a history of difficulties that predate other lupus symptoms, such as panic attacks in shops, fear of motorway driving or inability to travel in confined spaces like those on the Tube. Often the person will not have connected these symptoms with lupus.

- **Finger flexor tendonitis** Inflammation of the joints and tendons is one of the most common features of lupus. It may be possible for a doctor to identify this symptom when a patient cannot press the palms of their hands together – doctors refer to this as 'unable to say their prayers'. This condition is a useful pointer to lupus as it is subtly but significantly different in pattern from early rheumatoid arthritis, Lyme disease and other disorders.

- **Premenstrual symptoms** All rheumatic diseases are clinically influenced by the menstrual cycle, and this is particularly the case with lupus. Some people are almost immobilised during the two to three days preceding menstruation. A significant premenstrual flare is a strong indicator of lupus.

• **_Family history of autoimmune disease_** We now know that lupus is linked to your genes, so the presence of other autoimmune conditions in the family – including thyroid disease – is important.

'But you look so well'

The subject of the appearance of a person who has lupus is included here because it concerns a key characteristic of lupus, which can give confusing messages to those around you, thereby potentially affecting your diagnosis and treatment.

For many people with lupus the above heading will be all too familiar and unwelcome. It's an odd thing, but in the lupus clinic at St Thomas' Hospital people try not to say how well someone is looking – a simple pleasantry like that can be distressing to a patient because in lupus looks can be deceptive. One of the most annoying things about this condition is that unlike any other disease, it can actually give you the appearance of glowing health. You can look as though you have been sunning yourself in an exotic location, and you appear to be brimming with energy. Your cheeks may be rosy and your eyes sparkling. In fact, this is a nasty trick that lupus plays, because for many people with lupus the truth is that they might look as though they are well on the outside, but inside they feel as though they are dying. The fact that steroids tend to make your face fuller contributes to this look of well-being.

Those reading this who haven't had experience of lupus will think people who look good despite being ill should be grateful that they don't resemble the living dead. But there is a major problem when your looks are dramatically at odds with your state of health. When you look good no one really believes you can be so sick. It gives off a confusing message to those around you. We are all programmed to expect some visual confirmation that a person is very sick. It is easy to sympathise with someone who has a broken leg, for instance, or who has lost their hair because of chemotherapy.

In discoid lupus you can see the suffering as the rashes and red marks that are symptoms of the disease are often on areas of the body that are highly visible, like the face, neck or hands. Conversely, although SLE is the more life-threatening form of lupus, it shows little outward sign of its presence while doing damage within. Lupus is often referred to as a hidden disease not just because it is fickle and hard to pinpoint, but also because it is generally impossible to spot someone who has it just by looking at them.

When I was talking to people during the course of researching this book, the issue of appearance came up time and time again. Because lupus is difficult to diagnose in the first place, arriving in front of a GP looking fit and well will not help to impress upon them how sick you really are. Being doubted is one of the tougher aspects of lupus. If people don't believe you are ill then you won't get the treatment you need, nor the care and back-up that will help you cope.

That's not to say that lupus patients always look well. On the hospital wards where those in the throes of a violent flare are being treated, the evidence of the internal suffering becomes apparent. As the disease has taken hold and attacked major organs or connective tissue, or brought on the debilitating fatigue, patients lose the glow – but by then they are so sick that they couldn't care less how they look or who believes them.

If you are the one with lupus or someone who suspects they have lupus, don't be surprised if there are those around you who doubt the seriousness of your condition. If you are a family member or friend of a lupus sufferer, remember that looks can be deceptive. Listen to what the affected person says and don't dismiss their symptoms just because you cannot see them. The sick person needs to know they are believed and supported.

*   *   *

Having described the main general symptoms of lupus, the next chapter deals with related diseases – those that may occur simultaneously with lupus, and those that closely resemble lupus and may initially be mistaken for it. All this information will help you to gain an in-depth knowledge of your condition.

Chapter 4

Related Diseases

As if having lupus wasn't bad enough the reality is that it often comes with one or more other autoimmune problems. Now you might be fortunate enough to have just one disease, or one type of lupus but a high percentage of patients are found to have two or more conditions. For instance I have lupus, Raynaud's and scleritis – all are explained below. Autoimmune conditions can also mimic each other so the picture can be very confusing. This crossover of diseases is one of the reasons that lupus is so hard to diagnose and no one knows why a patient can have a parcel of autoimmune problems other than the fact that they have a dysfunctional immune system. It is up to the doctors to tackle this tricky area and reach the right diagnosis but as a patient it will help you to be aware of the most common conditions that overlap lupus or can appear to be SLE. What follows are brief descriptions of the diseases you might hear your doctor talk about. If you are told you have any of the following then you should ask for more details from your medical team.

You can have so many tongue twisters next to your name that you begin to feel like a medical oddity. When you recite your personal list of ailments it's embarrassing – you either laugh or end up crying. Laughter is always a tonic if you can manage it. When I think of the autoimmune conditions that I have it seems almost farcical. It brings to mind a sketch from the comedy series Blackadder where the main character Edmund, played by Rowan Atkinson, meets a jailor called Mr Ploppy who boasts of his collection of fascinating diseases.

Edmund: 'Ploppy, son of Ploppy the jailer?'

Mr Ploppy: 'Ah ach, no Sir. I am the first Ploppy to rise to be jailer. My father, Daddy Ploppy, was known as Ploppy the slopper. It was from him that I inherited my fascinating skin diseases.'

Edmund: 'Yes, you are to be congratulated, my friend. We live in an age where illness and deformity are commonplace and yet, Ploppy, you are without a doubt the most repulsive individual that I have ever met. I would shake your hand but I fear it would come off.'

Mr Ploppy: 'There's not many bosses would be that considerate, sir.'

Disorders that can be part of lupus

The following conditions can occur either as part of lupus, or on their own.

Hughes syndrome

This condition – which is also known as sticky blood, or antiphospholipid syndrome (APS) – is one of the most important recent discoveries in the field of autoimmunity. It is expected that it will become the most common autoimmune disease this century. It is more prevalent than multiple sclerosis (MS), rheumatoid arthritis, leukaemia or HIV, but because it is still new in medical terms it is relatively unknown. The condition was first identified by the medical consultant for this book, Dr Graham Hughes, in the early 1980s, and was originally called antiphospholipid syndrome, or APS, but was later renamed after Dr Hughes.

It was observed that there was a high incidence of miscarriage and blood clots among women with lupus. Further research showed that this was because the blood contained antiphospholipid antibodies that made it more viscous, or sticky, and therefore prone to excessive clotting. In pregnancy this can cause the fine capillaries in the placenta to become blocked, thereby limiting the vital blood supply to the foetus.

In the years that followed the initial discovery, research showed that Hughes syndrome was not limited to those with lupus. In fact, it was much more widespread than SLE, occurring in a wide cross-section of the population. One in three lupus patients test positive for this autoimmune condition, which can affect any part of the body.

A good analogy for Hughes syndrome is provided by the engine of a car. If the fuel in the car thickens the engine will not be able to function properly. It will begin to stutter and the vehicle can no longer run smoothly. This is what happens when someone has sticky blood. The condition affects veins and arteries, so it can cause clots in both. It is responsible for a fifth of recurrent miscarriages, strokes in young people and deep vein thrombosis (DVT). It can cause neurological problems such as speech and memory loss, as well as joint pain, fatigue and severe headaches.

Like lupus, Hughes syndrome can be difficult to diagnose because of ignorance about the condition. There are highly effective tests that have been developed to spot Hughes syndrome, but the key is knowing to ask for them. For instance, if you have had one or more miscarriages, any blood clots, a history of severe headaches, speech difficulties or memory problems, ask your doctor to test for this condition. The tests are widely available (*see page 69* for details of the tests).

If left untreated Hughes syndrome can do serious damage and can even be fatal. The better news is that if you test positive for the condition, it responds well to blood-thinning drugs. There are numerous cases where the right treatment can lead to dramatic reversals, in particular with regard to miscarriage. If you have Hughes syndrome and are being closely monitored you stand a good chance of having a successful pregnancy (*see page 132*).

Hughes syndrome affects men and women of any age – the ratio between the sexes is much closer than it is in lupus (*see page 127*), more like three women to one man in the period between puberty and middle age. People can have the condition without knowing it, or they can have suffered symptoms for years without being diagnosed due to ignorance of it.

Helen Pettitt, a fitness trainer, almost lost her life to this disease. She had suffered from sore joints since her early teens, which was particularly frustrating for someone who was a promising athlete. Helen ran for her local sports club. Despite repeated visits to the doctor the only diagnosis that was forthcoming was that she suffered from growing pains. Helen was given a mild analgesic and was left to cope with the soreness. It wasn't until she was twenty-six that she found out the hard way that she had a potentially fatal disease. In 1997, when she was backpacking in New Zealand, she became acutely ill.

I had a pain in my throat for two days before the heart attack. I was eating packets of throat lozenges because I thought I had an infection. I was in Auckland with my new boyfriend Andy. I resisted seeing a doctor, but one evening he said that if I wasn't better by the morning he would take me to the local hospital.

As it turned out I didn't make it through the night. It got to three o'clock in the morning and I fell to the floor. The pain was second to none; it felt as though I had swallowed a needle – two points digging in on either side of my throat. The pain in my chest felt as though someone had got a belt around it and was tightening it notch by notch. Andy got me in a cab to the hospital. They put me in a side room – they clearly thought I would be all right. After a while I sent Andy home because he doesn't like hospitals. Then I rang him at 7.30 in the morning as I was becoming more and more scared. The pain would come and go and get worse and worse. When he got there I lost all feeling down my left arm; I had pins and needles.

I couldn't feel anything but knew I was going to be sick and asked for something to be sick into. I saw the nurse walk out of the room and that was the last thing I remember. Andy said that at this stage I was almost fitting, I had passed out, and my lips were blue. The next thing I knew I was waking up in resus stark naked. I was told that Andy had been sent away as the crash team had cut my clothes off me to gave me three bursts of electricity. My heart had stopped beating. They said I had been dead for about three minutes.

My heart had stopped totally. I think it was a blood clot due to Hughes Syndrome. It took them a week of tests to find out what the problem was. A nurse came in and said, 'We've found out what's wrong with you.' It was such a relief. She said, 'You've got lupus and Hughes syndrome.' I had never heard of either. They described it as all these antibodies going around my body. There was more to come, though – they also found polycystic kidneys and no spleen.

Auckland Hospital was brilliant. What was staggering for me was that it took them just a week to find out what was wrong, whereas in England I had been ill for about fourteen years and totally in the dark. The staff photocopied all my files, and gave me Dr Graham Hughes' name. I'd had to go backpacking in New Zealand and have a heart attack to find out what was wrong with me.

These days I am much better. Andy and I are still together and we just get on with our lives.

Sjogren's syndrome

This is like a little brother to lupus. It can be present on its own or alongside lupus. The symptoms are similar, including joint pain, fatigue and mouth ulcers. The quite specific symptoms in Sjogren's involve the eyes and mouth becoming excessively dry. It's an autoimmune condition that attacks saliva glands in the body's mucous membranes – the soft linings around the eyes, genitals and mouth that secrete fluids to keep these areas well lubricated. As is the case with lupus, the vast majority of people affected are women, although with this condition 90 per cent of them are over the age of fifty-five.

The condition can be so mild that you hardly notice it and might not know you have it until tests show you do. Sometimes we unconsciously adjust to irritations like dry eyes or mouth without linking them to other symptoms, such as joint pain.

At the other end of the scale Sjogren's can be much more than an irritant. It can make your eyes so dry that blinking and eye movement is difficult. Your eyes can feel scratchy with a burning sensation, which happens especially in the mornings. You might also find that you cannot cope with bright light. One source of relief is to use artificial tears.

Your mouth can become very dry, making it difficult to swallow or even speak. If you have Sjogren's you may have to suck on special lozenges to give some lubrication.Another cause for concern is that the lack of saliva can lead to tooth decay and gum disease. Saliva normally helps protect the gums and teeth by lining them. It is important to let your dentist know if you have Sjogren's, and you must have regular check-ups to see if there is decay. One handy tip is to suck on bitter foods like lemons as they prompt the glands in the mouth to secrete saliva. Obviously it is important to brush and floss regularly when you have Sjogren's.

You should be aware that Sjogren's can cause vaginal dryness, which may make sexual intercourse uncomfortable or painful. There are lubricants available across the counter that can help, but you should let your doctor know if you are having problems.

Raynaud's phenomenon

People with lupus often have problems with extremes of temperature. Raynaud's is one manifestation of this and is common in lupus. If you have the disorder your fingers and toes turn red and then white quite suddenly, usually when exposed to the cold or stress. They can then turn bluish to black and feel numb and painful. This is because the fine blood vessels contract in the cold and cut off the blood flow. Less commonly, Raynaud's can also be seen in the feet, tongue, tip of the nose and outer part of the ears.

Shaking and massaging the affected body parts should bring back the feeling, although when the circulation finally returns they can throb and feel sore. There isn't really a treatment specifically for this condition; prevention is the best option – avoid the cold if you can. If not, then be prepared. Some people make sure they have thermal gloves available at all times – tucked away in pockets, bags and the car; thermal socks are also recommended. Others go so far as to use electrically heated gloves.

Fibromyalgia

Fibromyalgia affects about 20 per cent of people who have lupus. It is a separate condition and can be mistaken for lupus as some of the symptoms are similar – in particular the chronic fatigue. It is a syndrome that affects the muscles, making them very painful and weak. Like lupus, it is a fickle condition that can come and go, and can affect various parts of the body at different times. Fibromyalgia – which means painful muscles, tendons and ligaments – affects sleep patterns so that a person suffering from it will not be refreshed from sleep, waking up tired and stiff. They can have severe headaches and suffer from an irritable bowel, involving frequent diarrhoea or constipation with gut pain and nausea. Fibromyalgia can also lead to personality changes. People who have lupus and fibromyalgia can be highly sensitive to sunlight.

No one knows what causes this syndrome, or why there is a cross-over with lupus. In the treatment for fibromyalgia, analgesics are used to reduce pain and mild antidepressants are given to relax the person and help them get some sleep.

Myositis

Myositis, or dermatomyositis, is inflammation of the muscles, and it needs to be spotted early on to prevent serious damage. The first muscles to be affected are usually those nearer the centre of the body – the thighs, shoulders, neck, pelvis and upper arms. You might feel a burning sensation in your muscles, which will be followed by pain and subsequently weakness. Myositis is a cause for concern in lupus as it can do permanent harm. There are muscle-function tests that will check the strength of muscles by gauging the electrical impulses from them. Loss of muscle tone can also be caused by high-dose steroids.

It is important to spot any muscle damage early on so that measures can be taken to stop the deterioration. Treatment includes physiotherapy and a carefully monitored exercise regime to reverse any significant weakness.

Disorders that mimic lupus

These are disorders that are linked to lupus or can be mistaken for lupus, but are in fact not part of the condition.

Mixed connective tissue disease

You might find that after lots of tests your doctor says you have a form of lupus called mixed connective tissue disease (MCTD). To all intents and purposes MCTD is lupus, although there are some differences. MCTD is rarely life threatening – unlike SLE it does not attack major organs like the kidneys. The 'mixed' part of this name refers to the fact that someone may have some of the symptoms of lupus but also those of other diseases, including scleroderma (*see page 62*) and myositis (*see page 60*). There are four major features of MCTD:

- Raynaud's phenomenon – fingers turning white in the cold.
- Arthritis – obvious swelling of joints; fingers swollen like sausages.
- Unusual to have major kidney disease.

• The presence of a specific antibody – anti-RNP (anti-ribonucleoprotein).

Because MCTD is not as life threatening as lupus can be, the treatment is more conservative and the amount of medication needed is less. Still, MCTD does need to be monitored regularly to watch out for any aggressive changes.

Rheumatoid arthritis

The symptoms of rheumatoid arthritis are similar to those of lupus in that they involve the joints. It can be difficult to define which disease is present, especially in the early stages, although blood tests will help. It is unlikely that someone will have both conditions. There are some crucial differences between the two. Most importantly, rheumatoid arthritis can do permanent damage to the joints by eroding them, whereas lupus does not do actual damage and once the inflammation goes the joints usually function normally. On the reverse side is the fact that lupus can threaten major organs, whereas rheumatoid arthritis is only found in the joints.

Scleroderma

This condition can be mistaken for lupus in the early stages but it is actually a very different autoimmune condition. It is where the skin becomes thick – it looks hard, glossy and red. It is associated with Raynaud's phenomenon (*see page 59*), but is more severe. It can be confined to the hands and feet but in the majority of cases it slowly works its way up the body, changing the appearance of the skin on the arms, chest and even the mouth and nose. More worrying is when it attacks the internal organs. For instance, it can thicken the oesophagus, which carries food from the mouth to the stomach, and this can make swallowing difficult and uncomfortable.

Behcet's disease

This is a condition that is most commonly found in certain ethnic groups from the Mediterranean and Middle East, for instance Turkey, Iran and Iraq. It appears to be similar to lupus as it causes both mouth and genital ulcers. Those affected are also likely to have arthritis and problems with blood vessels. Despite the similarities the diseases are very different and blood tests will clearly define which one is present.

Rheumatic fever

This was once a common condition but better treatment and medication has resulted in it becoming rare in Western countries. The fever takes the form of an acute arthritis, which comes after a streptococcal throat infection. Blood tests are used to differentiate this condition from lupus.

Wegener's granulomatosis

This involves the inflammation of the blood vessels, but it is totally different from lupus. Wegener's is a rare and serious condition. It can make your nose run and feel stuffy, and you might find that you get a bloody nose. It involves a chronic thickening of the tissue of the sinuses in the forehead and behind the eyes. It becomes a particular cause for concern when it spreads to the lungs, causing coughing and breathing difficulties, and it can affect other organs in the body. Blood tests and clinical examination will help differentiate this condition from lupus. The use of cyclophosphamide is highly effective and can lead to remission.

Polyarteritis nodosa

Like Wegener's granulomatosis, this condition involves the inflammation of blood vessels but is very different from lupus. It is a dramatic inflammation of the major arteries, in particular in the legs, making it painful to walk. It can also affect major organs like the heart, and cause joint pains. It is life threatening, but if treated the symptoms are totally reversible. Again, blood tests and clinical examination will help to differentiate this condition from lupus.

The next chapter describes the types of test that are carried out to help establish the presence of lupus.

Chapter 5

Tests for Lupus

There is no one test for lupus. Specialists take a broad view on a patient-by-patient basis, because each person is different and the disease manifests itself in differing ways. Doctors consider various factors, including past and present symptoms, the medical history of the patient and their family, blood and other tests, and clinical observations. No one factor will lead to the diagnosis – a doctor will piece together the whole picture before concluding that lupus is the culprit.

Blood tests

One of the main ways of finding out if you have lupus is through blood tests. Over the years they have become more efficient as a means of spotting the antibodies that reveal the activity of this disease. There are numerous tests that your doctor might want to have done, and some are likely to be repeated at regular intervals – especially if you are having a flare – to keep an eye on how active the lupus is.

Antinuclear antibody (ANA) test

This test sounds like something out of an atomic science lab, but the 'nuclear' part refers to the nuclei found in all cells in the body. As explained in Chapter 1, in lupus the immune system goes haywire and produces antibodies that attack healthy cells and tissue. These are also known as autoantibodies, auto meaning 'self'. 'Antinuclear' means there are antibodies attacking the nuclei of the cells.

This test is regarded as the most sensitive one for establishing whether someone has lupus. A positive ANA will provide an indication that lupus is present, although it is not conclusive. ANA isn't only linked with lupus – a positive test can indicate the presence of other autoimmune diseases like Sjogren's syndrome, scleroderma or rheumatoid arthritis. ANA can be found in people who are healthy. This is why a positive ANA test cannot be used as the only diagnostic test for lupus.

Deoxyribonucleic acid (DNA) antibody test

DNA is found in the nucleus of a cell and provides the basic building blocks for a person's genetic make-up. This test looks at whether the DNA has been attacked by antibodies. It is carried out alongside ANA (see above) as it is much more specific to lupus. Research has shown that the antibodies attack the DNA of people with lupus. The test helps to eliminate other diseases, like rheumatoid arthritis, where the antibodies do not target DNA.

A positive DNA antibody test will be regarded as strong evidence that you have lupus. The levels of DNA antibodies will be measured regularly to get a feel for how aggressive the disease is. A rapidly rising presence of antibodies will set alarm bells ringing, while a drop will indicate that the condition is heading towards remission.

Extractable nuclear antigens (ENA) test

This group includes numerous antibodies found in lupus and other diseases connected with lupus, such as Sjogren's syndrome and mixed connective tissue disease. These antibodies are very useful to specialists as they can help define the type of disease activity.

The anti-Ro antibody, which is found in a quarter of people with lupus, is the most important in this group. It is regarded as an indicator that relatively mild lupus is present. Ro is the name given to a protein that exists in the fluid within the cell and can be seen in patients who have tested negative for antinuclear antibodies (*see page 66*). It is also associated with Sjogren's syndrome, as well as with photosensitivity, drug allergy and mild neurological problems like numbness.

There is a sinister aspect of the anti-Ro antibody, namely that in a tiny percentage of women it can pass to their children and create a risk of the cardiac condition known as heart block. It is therefore important for blood tests to be carried out to check if it is present. There is more about this in Chapter 9 (*see page 136*).

Anti-Sm antibodies test

Like the DNA antibodies test (*see page 66*), this test is specific to lupus. 'Sm' stands for Smith, who was the patient in whom this protein was first identified. Once again, a positive test will point to lupus but a negative result does not totally exclude the disease being present.

Erythrocyte sedimentation rate (ESR) test

You might hear your doctor talk about your 'ESR' being raised. This is a widely used blood test to establish if there is inflammatory activity in the body. ESR stands for erythrocyte sedimentation rate, which refers to the speed at which the red blood cells sediment to the bottom of a test tube The full name is rarely used – you might hear it called the 'sed' rate.

If there is inflammation in the body the ESR is raised. This test is therefore widely used as measure of inflammatory activity in the body. A normal ESR would be around 20 mm/hr (millimetres per hour); if it goes up to 100 mm/hr or more, there is likely to be a lot of inflammation. It could, however, be raised due to the flu or a vast array of other problems that have nothing to do with lupus. The test is thus rather crude and can be contradictory – for instance a person can have a normal ESR even though they are very ill, while others might always have a raised ESR when they don't appear unwell. Despite its limitations, this test is considered a useful clinical guide and can give an early indication that problems are occurring.

C-reactive protein (CRP) test

This is also a barometer of disease activity. It is the measurement of a protein or antibody released into the blood by the liver, which in general goes up dramatically with acute inflammation. In lupus, however, this is not the case – the odd thing is that the CRP does not rise if the disease is present. If, therefore, a person is found to have a high ESR but a normal CRP, then it increases the possibility that they have lupus.

Complement test

Your doctor might order a 'complement' test. Complements are a group of proteins found in the blood and are linked to the way the immune system functions. The various proteins in this group are identified by using the letter 'C' followed by a number, and the most commonly measured proteins in lupus are C3 and C4. If they are low and the levels are falling, this is regarded as a clear warning that a flare is imminent or under way, as the complement is being used up during disease activity.

Full blood screen

Because of advances in blood-testing procedures it is often cheaper and quicker just to order up a full blood screen. This means looking at white and red blood cell levels, platelet count, liver and kidney function, haemoglobin, calcium and cholesterol. If there are abnormalities in any of these areas this will help a doctor piece together the evidence for or against lupus being present. In lupus the kidney function is of particular importance and an abnormal blood test might be the first indication that damage is being done. As mentioned earlier (*see page 42*), the attack on the kidneys is 'silent', so you might not know that something is wrong.

Antiphospholipid antibodies and lupus anticoagulant tests

There are two specific tests to determine whether you have Hughes syndrome (*see page 54*). The anticardiolipin antibody test – referred to as aCL – measures the amount of antiphospholipid antibodies in the blood. It is these antibodies that make the blood more viscous, or thick, and therefore more likely to clot.

The second test, known as lupus anticoagulant, is carried out in tandem with aCL as there are slight differences between them and some people can test positive for one and not the other. The name lupus anticoagulant is, however, misleading, as this is not a test for lupus.

Other tests

Urine tests

The silent nature of kidney involvement makes urine tests very important and people with lupus should have them done regularly. Some clinics teach patients how to do their own dipstick test to check for blood or proteins. This test is essential, as lupus attacks the kidneys, but as mentioned (*see page 42*) symptoms can be few in the early stages so a patient may not even know that there is a problem in this area.

Scans

X-rays were never detailed enough to give a clear picture of lupus disease activity, especially in the brain. Today there are two types of scan that allow doctors to see much more clearly what is going on. These are the computed tomography (CT) scan and the magnetic resonance imaging (MRI) scan. You may find the idea of having a scan a bit daunting, but neither type of scan is painful or particularly uncomfortable.

If you are having a CT scan you will usually be asked to lie very still on a pallet as a large scanner, shaped like a white halo around the pallet, moves along your body to the area that needs scanning. You might have an injection of iodine, which doesn't hurt but feels warm as it passes around your body – this will just be to help define the area being examined.

When you have a MRI scan you also lie on a pallet. You might be given a small buzzer to hold in your hand just in case you want to stop the test. The pallet moves into a tube-like chamber that completely surrounds your body, or if only your brain is being scanned they may just move your head into the chamber. There will be plenty of space around you, although you might feel a bit claustrophobic. The staff are well used to reassuring patients. If you do feel anxious they might decide to give you a mild sedative while the procedure is under way. There is an intercom in the chamber that you can use to talk to the medical staff and let them know if you are having problems. You'll be asked to keep still as the scan is carried out. Don't be alarmed by lots of loud clicking and banging – that will just be part of the machine doing its job.

In lupus, the MRI scan is used mostly to check if the disease has affected the brain. It will show up lesions or blood clots, which will appear as white blobs on the scan picture. The clarity of these test results has provided doctors with a highly effective tool to spot damage, although the scan should not be used in isolation to reach a diagnosis.

Biopsy

Sometimes it is necessary to go right to the heart of the problem to find out what is going on. A biopsy is a test where tissue or cells are removed from the body so that they can be examined more closely for disease activity. Most biopsies are minor procedures that are done using a local anaesthetic, although they can be more invasive if a doctor wants to check the condition of major organs like the kidneys. In some cases you may have to have a biopsy done under a general anaesthetic.

Shirmer's test

This is a simple but highly useful test for Sjogren's syndrome (*see page 58*), which involves using strips of specially prepared blotting paper a few millimetres long. These are placed on the lower eyelid, which feels a bit scratchy but is otherwise painless. The normal reaction to such an irritant would be the production of fluid from the duct and the paper would become soaked in a matter of seconds. In someone with Sjogren's, however, the paper will remain bone dry even if you wait for a number of minutes. Despite the fact that this is an inexpensive test it isn't often carried out at GP level, which is a shame. If a doctor suspects autoimmune problems in someone with joint inflammation and fatigue, doing a Shirmer's test might save time and help get an early diagnosis for Sjogren's or lupus.

Chapter 6

The Four
Main Treatments

It can be a scary moment when your doctor comes to the
end of your appointment and begins to scribble madly on
lots of multi-coloured bits of paper. The only things you
recognise are the stickers on each document with your
name and hospital number on them. As you walk out of
the room heading towards the pharmacy with a wedge of
paperwork, you probably won't have much of an idea what
the medications are – especially if you are new to lupus.

The doctor should have explained what you are being
given, how the drugs work and how much to have of each
one and when. Even then it can be a lot to take in. No one
likes swallowing pills, and in lupus you can find yourself
having to take so many that you leave the chemist with a
carrier bag full! There is, however, compelling evidence that
in this disease drugs are required for survival. This is certainly
the case at crucial stages, for instance during an aggressive
flare, especially where major organs are under attack.

More than 90 per cent of people with lupus are on some
form of medication at any one time. That doesn't mean to
say you will be popping pills all your life. As specialists get
better at tweaking doses to keep them low, and as drugs

become more sophisticated, there is an increasing chance that lupus sufferers can look forward to a day that will start with just a cup of tea, and not having to use it to wash down a handful of pills. The catch is that to get to that point you have to take your medicine. Work to refine the more toxic drugs is under way, and new products are always in the pipeline.

A key advance is in the way the drugs are used. Doctors today have moved away from 'using hammers to crack nuts'. Instead they look closely at the balance of the medications. It is rather like working out a recipe; a teaspoonful of this, a few milligrams of that, with an injection of the other. Tinkering with dosage sizes like this takes a great deal of expertise, but it isn't only the province of the doctors; there are plenty of experienced patients who have learned how to adjust their dosages to suit themselves. This close monitoring of drug use can save a patient from unpleasant side effects and the clinical evidence shows that it is just as effective as 'mega-dosing'.

If we take the example of steroids, for instance, twenty years ago everyone with lupus was poisoned with them. You would see people developing Cushing's syndrome, where their faces would be moon-shaped, and they would become obese and have osteoporosis, with weakened, crumbling bones. People would be on doses of 60 to 80 mg a day as a matter of routine, and anyone whose condition displayed central nervous system involvement would be put on 100 mg a day. They would balloon in size within days, develop mental problems and have disturbed sleep patterns, and their muscles would become very weak. The side effects of high-dose steroids were horrendous. It was the team at St Thomas' Hospital who helped push for low-dose steroids in lupus.

Today the recognition of the fact that if you control the disease carefully you can come out at the other end and get off medicines is vital. Lupus patients often don't believe specialists who tell them that they can look forward to a day without the pills. They don't think it will happen, but it does.

What's in a name?

One major area that causes confusion lies in how doctors refer to medications. The same drug can appear to have a number of different names. In actual fact, it doesn't. Each medication has a chemical or generic name and is then given a trade name by the drug company producing it. There can be several different trade names for the same drug, as certain medications are produced by a number of pharmaceutical firms. You can see a variation of the two names on prescriptions and notes. It helps to remember that the trade name will always start with a capital letter whereas the generic one won't. The difference in names is particularly noticeable in different countries. For instance, in Britain Brufen is the name commonly given to ibuprofen, whereas in the US it becomes Motrin.

People are often puzzled when they see steroids referred to variously as 'prednisone' or 'prednisolone'. In fact, these are the most widely used steroids in the world and are virtually the same. Prednisone is converted to prednisolone in the body by the liver. If in doubt ask your doctor what the chemical and trade names are for your drugs and make a note of them so that you will be familiar with them in future.

The big 'four'

Although you may be prescribed a large number of prescription drugs, four main types of medication are generally used in lupus. These are:

- Antimalarials.
- Non-steroidal anti-inflammatory drugs (NSAIDs).
- Immunosuppressives.
- Steroids.

You can have adverse reactions to any drugs. In rare cases, for instance, people are allergic even to low-dose aspirin. Some of the drugs used in lupus are powerful and the long lists of possible side effects can be frightening. It is important to understand the risk with medications. That way you can make a more informed decision about what you take. You also have to remember that any side effects are generally reversible and you might have to put up with them in order to get through a flare. Remember also that the list of side effects is not linked to the frequency with which they can occur. There is a good chance that you will escape any problems.

Your doctor will not just dish out toxic drugs without carefully weighing up how great your need is compared with the possible risk of taking the medication. If you do have concerns let the doctor know – it might be that there is an alternative drug that suits you better.

Antimalarials

The clue to this drug is in its name. This range of medication was initially developed to protect people against malaria. If you have visited the tropics you are likely to have been given a course of antimalarials to take to protect you from this parasitic disease, which is spread by the bites of the anopheles mosquito. The basic drug is called chloroquine.

St Thomas' Hospital led the way in the use of antimalarials in lupus. About a hundred years ago Dr Payne, a dermatologist at St Thomas', published a report detailing how effective they had been in combating discoid or skin lupus. He also noted that they helped resolve symptoms like fever and joint pain. This was supported by evidence that came to light during the Second World War. British troops stationed in the Pacific were given antimalarials. They were on the drug for a number of years and army medics started hearing reports from men who had arthritis or skin lesions that their conditions had cleared up. This led to further research, which was published in the *Lancet* in 1951; it clearly showed that antimalarials were effective in the treatment of conditions like rheumatoid arthritis and lupus.

What the research didn't show was why the drug worked – another of the great raft of medical mysteries linked with lupus. However, perhaps the 'why' isn't as important as the fact that this discovery has provided a highly effective and safe treatment for milder forms of lupus. Antimalarials are a steroid-sparing medication. It is thought that they suppress the immune system and they have an antiviral effect. They also partially block ultraviolet light – which is good for those with lupus who are very sun sensitive. Antimalarials are a mild anti-clotting agent, which helps those people who suffer from Hughes syndrome (*see page 54*).

As there are so few side effects and the doses are low, many lupus specialists keep patients on antimalarials for years. There are several products in this range of drugs, but the one you are likely to be given is called Plaquenil. Its chemical name is hydroxychloroquine. There are also Nivaquine and Atabrine, but both of these are less favoured by doctors as they can cause more side effects. Plaquenil is likely to be one of the first medications that you are prescribed. As it works slowly, it can take three months to kick in, but over the long term the evidence is strong that it slows down the disease.

Plaquenil is known to be effective in a number of areas. It reduces fatigue and fever, is very effective for skin lesions and is a good anti-inflammatory, easing joint and muscle pain, and helping to reduce mouth ulcers and hair loss. Antimalarials can have a dramatic effect on skin lupus, sometimes clearing up severe rashes in a matter of weeks. The usual dose is between one 200 mg tablet and two 400 mg tablets a day. In some cases a doctor might introduce two types of antimalarial to bring bad discoid lupus under control.

If you are heading off to a tropical area and need protection from mosquitoes, you will need to discuss this with your doctor as the Plaquenil you are taking for lupus will not give you full protection against malaria.

Side effects

In general antimalarials are very safe drugs. The usual low dosage results in side effects being kept to a minimum, but they can still cause problems in some people. The one that concerns doctors the most is the possible impact on your eyes. In the past, large doses of hydroxychloroquine led to problems with the retina, leading to visual disturbances and even blindness. It is now recognised that hydroxychloroquine is far far less likely than chloroquine to affect the eyes. A study at St Thomas' Hospital, of patients taking Plaquenil continuously for five years, showed there were no cases of problems with the eyes. It is nonetheless advisable to have an eye check before you start taking antimalarials, so that there is a baseline to measure any changes against, just in case. It is also recommended that you have an annual eye check.

Antimalarials can upset your stomach; you may feel

bloated and lose your appetite. Diarrhoea is a rare side effect. If you have any of these problems you must let your doctor know. It could be that the dose needs to be lowered or that you simply cannot tolerate the drug and have to stop taking it.

A word about pregnancy and Plaquenil: women used to be advised to stop this medication when they were pregnant. It is now known that hydroxychloroquine can be safely taken during this time, and in fact there is some evidence that when women stop taking the drug when they are pregnant, they run the risk of suffering a lupus flare.

For most people, antimalarials are free of side effects and over the long term can be highly effective in the control of lupus, especially in preventing further flares.

Non-steroidal anti-inflammatory drugs (NSAIDs)

NSAIDs have been developed as the next generation after aspirin in the treatment of arthritic problems. Up until thirty years ago high-dose aspirin was the only treatment available and that had lots of nasty side effects like ringing in the ears (also known as tinnitus), drowsiness and stomach problems. In fact, NSAIDs are less toxic than the high doses of aspirin were. They are used for pain and inflammation in lupus and are 'steroid sparing'. Some of the names for them you might come across are Feldene, Naprosyn, Voltarol, Relifex and Oruvail, although there are many more currently on the market and their names differ from country to country. There is so much choice within this group of medications that it can be a case of trial and error to find the right drug for you with the least side effects. NSAIDs work by stopping the production of enzymes that play a part in causing inflammation and pain.

Although you can switch between NSAIDs if you do not react well to them, it is worth giving each one a month or so before deciding whether it is the one for you, since it can take that long for the drug to become effective. This range of medications can be used in conjunction with another drug – like steroids – or on their own. NSAIDs are particularly useful for people with mild lupus, where major organs are not threatened. They can work well on reducing inflammation in joints and muscles.

Side effects

That is not to say that NSAIDs are free of side effects. The most common problem is with indigestion or an irritable gut. They can also lead to bleeding in the stomach or ulcers, especially in older people. If you have had a history of gastric problems you must make sure your doctor is aware of this. One way of keeping an eye on any possible bleeding is to have your blood count checked for anaemia. There are medications that can help line the gut to prevent bleeding – ranitidine (Zantac) or Losec work well. You might need antacids, and it is best to take the medication with food. There are new NSAIDs that have been developed to avoid damage to the stomach. Three of these are called Vioxx, Celebrex and Arcoxia, and they are proving to be highly effective.

You may find that your blood pressure goes up when you are taking NSAIDs because they can cause fluid retention – although this is rare. The kidneys can also be affected by this, so this is another area that has to be closely monitored. If you have had lupus nephritis and there is already some damage to the kidneys, it is not advisable for you to take NSAIDs.

Immunosuppressives

As I explained earlier (*see page 5*), lupus is a condition where the immune system has gone a bit mad, racing off into overdrive and attacking healthy parts of the body. Simple logic would tell you that one way of tackling this problem is to try and bring the system under control. Immunosuppressives do just that – they dampen the whole thing down, switching it off to some extent. Some of these drugs were in fact developed to help in organ transplants as a way of preventing the immune system from rejecting new organs, while others are used to treat cancer patients, so don't be surprised if you have heard of some of them in a different context.

Immunosuppressives are used by a high percentage of people with lupus, and in particular in cases where the disease is relatively aggressive and is threatening major organs and doctors have to work fast to prevent damage from being done. These are toxic drugs, however, and the more powerful ones come with their own selection of possible side effects (see below under individual drugs). It boils down to making a deal with the devil – if you are very sick and the doctors believe you need these drugs to survive, then the answer to the question of whether you should take them or not is straightforward.

Doctors use a number of different names for this category of medications. You might hear them call it chemotherapy, which is scary because of the association with cancer treatments. Or they could say they are going to give you cytotoxic drugs – these chemicals are designed to kill abnormal cells although they are toxic so they can kill healthy cells as well. (Cyto means cell and toxic means damage.) A much easier name to swallow is 'steroid-sparing', and that is exactly what they are – they can be used either instead of steroids or alongside them to lower the dose of steroids and thereby limit side effects. As in the case of steroids, the plan is always to use these strong drugs to bring the lupus under control, to stop irreparable damage being done to the body and then get patients off them. If you are on any of the immunosuppressives, you are advised to drink a lot of water to help flush the toxins out of the body.

Azathioprine

Azathioprine, or Imuran, is one of the most commonly used immunosuppressives. It is the one with the least side effects. It is often used in conjunction with steroids, so there is a balance between both drugs, with the aim of limiting the steroid. It can take time for azathioprine to kick in, so it is generally used for longer periods of time to prevent new flares and help keep the lupus in check. It is often used for milder kidney disease, or where it is proving difficult to drop the steroid dose.

People can be on azathioprine for a number of years without any adverse effects. That's not to say it doesn't have side effects. The most common is nausea. Some people just can't stomach the drug, and it makes them sick and takes away their appetite. In such cases, a doctor will consider a different immunosuppressive. Azathioprine can affect the liver or lead to a drop in the white blood cell count, and both these areas need to be closely monitored. When you are first put on azathioprine you will have a blood test to check that your liver is functioning properly and that your white blood cells are normal. This will be followed up at regular intervals.

Cyclophosphamide

Cyclophosphamide (Cytoxan) is the next most commonly used immunosuppressive drug. It is stronger than azathioprine. It is an effective drug which is used when lupus is threatening major organs or when it is affecting the brain and causing severe psychiatric problems. There has been a great deal of progress in recent years, so much so that doses have fallen and thereby side effects are limited. It used to be given orally in a tablet form but that lead to unpleasant side effects like cystitis. Now most lupus centres give it as an intermittent injection. At St Thomas' lupus clinic they will give 500 mg each week for three weeks and after that a monthly injection for six months or so. This is used in conjunction with a drug called Mesna which stops any irritation of the bladder.

Cyclophosphamide can reduce white blood cell count and when used in higher doses it can lead to infertility – affecting the ovaries or male sperm count. Because of the lessened immunity it can lead to virus infections or shingles. For people with serious kidney inflammation this is a wonder drug. Figures show that before it was used 75% of people with lupus nephritis - inflamed kidneys - would lose the use of those organs within five years, even with steroids. That is no longer the case. A key benefit of the new low dose regime is that it has dramatically cut the number of patients who become infertile. At St Thomas' the use of a low-dose cyclophosphamide amongst women in recent years has resulted in no cases of ovarian failure.

Methotrexate

This is used to get joint inflammation under control and has few side effects. It is now the world's most widely used medication in the treatment of severe rheumatoid arthritis. There is also some evidence that it can help in discoid lupus.

Steroids

Steroids are the main treatment for lupus flares. In recent years they have had a bad press, perhaps because of athletes using anabolic steroids to illegally boost performance, or due to the nasty side effects suffered by those on them for medical reasons. The bottom line is that steroids, which are also called corticosteroids, rank alongside aspirin as a miracle drug of modern times. In lupus they are a lifesaver as they are the most effective anti-inflammatory drugs available.

Steroids are remarkably quick and effective in reversing the swelling caused by autoimmunity. Most importantly, they deal with inflammation that threatens major organs, and also relieve the pain and tenderness that people with lupus experience. Explaining how they actually work is complex, but put in simple terms steroids help to make certain cells in the blood more stable, so that they are less likely to become involved in causing inflammation. Steroids also lower the number of lymphocytes, which are the main white blood cells of the immune system that play a big part in causing autoimmune problems.

The existence and benefits of steroids in medicine were first spotted by Dr Phillip Hench, an American rheumatologist working at the Mayo Clinic in the US in the 1930s and 1940s. He noticed that the arthritic pain and inflammation in certain patients would be resolved during pregnancy or if they had jaundice. This led to the discovery that natural hormones, or steroids, worked against pain and swelling. Dr Hench was awarded a Nobel prize for this remarkable discovery, which revolutionised the treatment of arthritic conditions, among many others.

Steroids were first used to deal with inflammation caused by lupus in the 1950s, and have been used ever since as one of the main drugs to treat SLE. What has changed dramatically over the past fifty years is how steroids are administered. The first generation of patients who were on large doses had serious problems with crumbling bones or furred arteries, but without them these people would not have survived. Lower doses in recent years have helped cut the severity and the number of people displaying these complications . . .

How much?

As Dr Hench found, the body makes its own supply of steroids (cortisone) in the adrenal glands. This hormone plays an important role in many bodily functions, in particular in preventing inflammation. When a person is given synthetically produced steroids the adrenal glands can decide that they don't need to keep making steroids so they 'close down'. Anyone starting on a course of steroids will therefore be repeatedly told not to suddenly stop taking them as this could leave their body without steroids, which could be life threatening.

Most doctors will adjust the dose in line with the condition of the patient. When someone is extremely ill they can take doses as high as 40 to 60 mg or more until the disease activity is under control, after which the dose is gradually lowered. Once a person has recovered and the inflammation is under control, the doctor will endeavour to bring the amount taken down to the body's natural level of steroid. This is a crucial stage in the control of lupus, because doctors find that dropping below 7.5 mg to 5 mg can either trigger another flare, or a patient can move to getting off the drug completely. It is a case of fine-tuning the dose prescribed, for example by reducing the dose by 1 mg a month. A doctor can also get a patient to take prednisolone on alternate days – say two 5 mg tablets on one day, followed by one the next, or have one day on and one day off them. The belief is that this can help the adrenal glands return to normal function and gives an indication of whether the lupus is likely to flare again – if the disease is still active, then a lower dose will lead to a return of the symptoms.

Steroids are also sometimes given as an injection, drops or creams. The aim is to use them 'topically', which means applying them directly to the area where they are needed and thereby limiting the side effects. 'Pulse' steroids are very high doses that are given intravenously – or directly into the vein – using a drip. This is a highly effective method of treatment for people who are acutely ill in hospital, or where a person has difficulty taking steroids orally. It is also used in cases where someone is able to get to a clinic but is in the middle of an aggressive flare – in particular where major organ damage to the kidneys or brain is involved – and needs a hefty 'quick fix'.

Pulse therapy usually lasts an hour and involves the person taking between 500 mg and 1000 mg methylprednisolone. The effects of pulse therapy can last for weeks or months. Steroids can be injected into muscles or joints to hit a target quickly, especially where someone is in extreme pain. This isn't something that is done time and again, though, as repeated injections over the long term can do some damage to cartilage.

Side effects

The main question asked by patients who are on steroids is 'What are the side effects?' Crucial to this is the fact that the lower the dose the fewer problems there are. People on a low dose, say 7.5 mg a day, are generally trouble free, especially if they are taking the steroids for a short period of time. For instance, if you are on steroids for roughly a month you are highly unlikely to suffer any adverse effects.

Before you read on, please let me give you a word of

warning. When you go through the information below do not despair. The chances are that you may get none of these complications, or perhaps only have them mildly. It is important to repeat that doctors now work hard to keep the doses as low as possible while still controlling the lupus. The other thing to remember is that once you are off the steroids most of the side effects tend to disappear quite quickly.

How you look

Steroids can affect how you look in a number of ways. One of the most noticeable and distressing side effects can be weight gain. This might appear to be nothing more than a cosmetic issue, but for people with lupus it is very hard to cope with – not only are you sick, but also you are putting on weight. Steroids give you the 'munchies', increasing your appetite and with that your waistline. To compound matters you will probably feel so unwell that exercise will be either out of the question or just something you really don't want to even think about. Also, because steroids are essentially based on male sex hormones, you can find (if you are a woman) that fat in your body is redistributed, for instance to your upper back, buttocks or stomach, with a subsequent thinning of the legs and arms. Then there is the 'moon face'. It is quite common for people to notice after a few weeks of taking steroids that their cheeks have puffed up like those of a hamster stocking up for winter. Facial hair in women can coarsen and become more prevalent. Steroids can also cause acne, or the skin can become more sensitive and prone to bruising. You may also find that cuts take longer to heal and that skin ulcers develop.

Before you rush for the paper bag to put over your head remember that it is likely that you won't have these problems. If you do, then comfort yourself with the knowledge that most of these side effects reverse within days or weeks either once your dose is lowered to around 7.5 mg, or when you get off the steroids altogether.

There are a few things you can do to alleviate the symptoms. Obviously, exercise is a good idea if you are up to it – swimming in particular as it supports your joints by lessening body weight. If you are suffering from increased appetite, try to keep an eye on what you are eating, and have healthy snacks like fruits and vegetables to hand. Because of the fluid retention avoid too much salt – a low-sodium, low-carbohydrate and low-calorie diet should help. It may be that you find you have oedema, which is swelling around your ankles, fingers and face due to water retention. There are diuretics that can help with this, but it is best to ask your specialist before taking this kind of medication.

Osteoporosis

Osteoporosis is the thinning of the bones. With this condition, the bones become brittle and weak and more likely to fracture. This is a natural process in people as they get older, and in general over the age of seventy about a third of the skeleton's density has diminished. There are, however, factors that can bring on osteoporosis earlier in life. It is much more common in women than in men, in particular after the menopause, when the ovaries no longer produce the oestrogen that is needed to help maintain bone mass.

The use of synthetic steroids can also cause osteoporosis as they limit the amount of calcium absorbed by the gut. Calcium is essential for healthy bones. People who are taking steroids are therefore monitored closely to assess the possible impact of steroids on their bones. They are often given a DEXA scan that measures bone density, which is followed up with further scans over the years to check for any adverse impact. A doctor will often prescribe calcium tablets with the steroids to try to protect the bones by increasing calcium intake.

Osteoporosis can also be found in those who are inactive and do not take regular exercise, or those who have had prolonged bed rest. One of the best ways to prevent or limit osteoporosis is to take regular exercise and ensure that your diet includes calcium and Vitamin D.

There are medications available that help protect the bones, such as bisphosphonates, which are synthetic substances that are said to coat the bones and protect them from disintegration. If you are worried about having brittle bones, talk to your doctor about it.

Behaving oddly

Taking high doses of steroids can make you feel and behave oddly. Those affected in this way can become moody and irritable, might feel agitated, and may have problems concentrating and get easily confused. In extreme cases they can suffer from psychosis – a mental disorder where a person loses touch with reality. Memory can also be affected. On the other hand, steroids can make you feel 'high'. Some people talk about feeling euphoric one minute and sinking to the depths of depression the next. If you are having violent mood swings, you must tell your doctor so that the dose of steroid can be adjusted to limit this side effect. Steroids can also disturb sleep patterns – they may cause someone to sleep all day and be awake all night, or result in them not sleeping at all. This can lead to chronic fatigue and depression. Mild sedatives may be prescribed to help with sleep as it is such a crucial part of managing lupus.

It is important to look out for these effects, and to be aware that you are unlikely to be going mad if you are experiencing them. The culprit for your strange feelings and behaviour is likely to be the steroids you are taking.

These problems will be resolved once the dose of the drug is changed or you come off it.

It is also important that the families of people who are taking steroids take these behaviour changes on board and realise that they are probably related to the drugs. The best way to help is to try to understand what changes are occurring. Family members must try to be supportive and not dismissive. If they accompany the person who is taking the drugs when they go to see their doctor, they can hear for themselves that the changes are drug induced and not a worrying new aspect of their loved one's character.

And the rest . . .

There are several other side effects that you need to be aware of. These are summarised below; if you suffer from any of them you must let your medical team know as soon as possible.

- Steroids can tickle up a pre-existing gut problem, like a peptic ulcer. If you have a history of gastric complications tell your doctor as there are medications that can help line the gut and protect it. They generally have no side effects. There are also prednisolone pills that come coated – they are usually red. Ask for these when the prescription is written. Try to take them with food.

- Muscle weakness is another common side effect. People who are on high doses of steroids for long periods can find it difficult to walk and in extreme cases have to use a wheelchair.

- Joints can be affected. They may become soft and contribute to mobility problems. In some cases this can lead to a condition known as 'avascular necrosis'. This is where a lack of circulation to certain joints leads to bone death, in particular in the shoulders, knees and hips. The increased fat released into the blood as a result of the steroids clogs up pathways to the bone, stopping blood supply. This condition is very painful as it makes movement of the damaged joints extremely difficult. Joint replacement may be necessary to alleviate the pain and regain mobility, but early detection should help prevent this from happening.

- Steroids can cause glucose intolerance and that means raised blood sugar, which in some cases can lead to diabetes.

- Eyesight may be affected. Steroids may increase pressure in the eyes, which can lead to glaucoma, and if they are used over a long period of time cataracts can form. If you think this might be a problem, get your eyes checked every six months or so.

- The increased level of fats in the blood – cholesterol – can contribute to a narrowing of the blood vessels, which is known as arteriosclerosis. This can have the knock-on effect of putting stress on the heart. The long-term use of steroids can therefore lead to cardiac problems, even heart attacks, so it is important to keep an eye on cholesterol levels in the blood. Once again, prevention is the best way of dealing with this – a balanced diet and exercise will help.

- People who are on steroids are more prone to infection than those who are not as their immune systems are not working normally. The steroids get in the way of some of the body's protective mechanisms that would normally kill invading elements like bacteria and viruses. Because of this, those who are taking steroids are advised to avoid people with infections like coughs and colds.

Steroids and children

Although lupus isn't seen as a disease that often affects young children, there is growing evidence that it could be more common than is currently thought. As doctors become more aware that lupus can appear in children, so the number of cases grows. This is dealt with in more detail in Chapter 10 (*see page 142*). In children steroids are also the main treatment for a flare – the treatment in general is actually similar to that given to adults. There is, however, evidence that steroids can stunt growth. This is a cause for concern and influences doctors to minimise the use of these drugs on children as much as possible.

Chapter 7

Specific Treatments

The previous chapter dealt with what doctors regard as the 'mainstream' medications, the drugs that are mostly regarded as 'big hitters', the ones they generally prescribe to deal with lupus. There is no doubt with this condition that they are lifesavers and are a necessary part of managing your health in lupus. But there are other drugs and treatments that are on the periphery but are still part of the lupus picture. For instance having hypertension or high blood pressure is something that is common in the general population, as a lupus patient your blood pressure will be monitored closely so hypertension will show up and if it is consistently high it will need treatment. You can also develop hypertension as a result of kidney problems or excessive weight gain – both seen in SLE.

Something for the skin

Discoid and cutaneous lupus rashes can be very sore, irritating and disfiguring. As they are often on parts of the body that are exposed, sufferers have to deal with the embarrassment as well as the discomfort. As mentioned earlier (*see page* 77) a number of the main medications used to treat systemic lupus can resolve skin problems. It might be, however, that you only suffer from discoid lupus – about 20 per cent of those who have lupus fall into this category. The good news is that the drugs you need are milder, or the doses will be lower.

Steroid-based creams and ointments

Antimalarials, oral steroids and immunosuppressives, taken internally, are used for discoid lupus, but creams and ointments are also an option. You can buy some steroid-based creams over the counter from a chemist, or obtain a stronger version on prescription from your doctor. Excessive use of steroid cream can actually damage the skin by making it thinner, so it is important to consult your doctor rather than simply going it alone.

Sunscreens

The key with skin lupus is to catch it early – if you suffer from it, you can become familiar with the initial signs of a rash developing. If you leave the disc-like sores they can blister and burst, possibly leaving permanent scarring that is red, scaly and thick. Prevention is the best way of tackling this aspect of lupus, so buy a strong sunscreen with a high sun-protection factor (SPF). Make sure you apply plenty of lotion often on exposed areas of your skin, and don't forget the places you might otherwise overlook, like the neck, the backs of your hands, the tops of your feet, the ears and the temples – these are often missed and are particularly affected by lupus. You can also get make-up with a strong SPF added. It sounds obvious, but if your scalp is involved, especially if you have suffered from alopecia, or hair loss, then you should wear a hat. All the usual warnings about sunbathing should be followed even more closely by people with lupus skin problems. Avoid the sun between 10 a.m. and 4 p.m., as this is when the ultraviolet rays are the strongest, cover up and avoid sunbeds.

Where the skin has been badly damaged and such damage is highly visible, for instance on the face, doctors might advise that the person has plastic surgery to disguise the scarring.

Thalidomide

Thalidomide is one of the most notorious drugs of all time. The damage it did to babies back in the 1950s and 1960s, who were born without limbs, still haunts people's memories. In recent years, however, thalidomide has been rehabilitated. Medical science has taken another look at it and is putting this medication to good use – it is, for instance, used in the treatment of certain forms of cancer, HIV and leprosy.

Thalidomide is also proving to be highly effective in controlling discoid lupus. Trials that have been run at St Thomas' Hospital show that thalidomide can work well to reverse severe cases of skin lesions. Because of its chequered history there are stringent controls in place to prevent the drug from being used by women who could become pregnant, and it is also not given to men who want to start a family.

The work at St Thomas' has shown that thalidomide can help to clear up discoid lupus 75 per cent of the time. The drawback is that it produces a high incidence of side effects, in particular damage to the nerves, some of it permanent. It can cause what is called a peripheral neuropathy, which is numbness and tingling that is felt in your fingers, hands, toes, feet and lips. It is still early days in the use of thalidomide in lupus and research is still under way, but the results are so promising that doctors are beginning to consider thalidomide as a frontline treatment rather than something to be used as a last resort.

Mary Baker, a successful businesswoman, has had a lifetime of coping with SLE. Her first flare came after the birth of her son Paul more than twenty years ago, but she didn't develop discoid lupus until 1999. Over the years Mary has become an expert on lupus. She has learned how to listen carefully to her body, reading the signs and recognising when treatment is needed. She says thalidomide is by far the best thing for the discoid lupus, and calls it her 'miracle drug':

> When the discoid lupus suddenly appeared a few years ago I didn't know what it was. I had sores all over my back, like ringworm. They would blister and then bleed. They spread up my back, onto my neck and ears and then my face. It was so bad that they wanted to take pictures of me – lovely. I have found that if I don't catch it early the discoid can become quite bad. I have had the blisters in my hair, in my eyes and on my face, and it is when it gets on my face that I do something about it. I don't care if it is on the rest of my body. Thalidomide is the only drug that touches the discoid, and for me it is a miracle cure. I have learned how to control the medication so I use only what I need to stop the blisters in their tracks. As soon as I feel them coming on I take thalidomide. It's brilliant and I have no side effects.

Dealing with raised blood pressure

It is important to keep a close eye on blood pressure particularly in lupus, where it can be raised as a result of damage to the kidneys. Some medications can also raise your blood pressure. A very high blood pressure will set medical alarm bells ringing as it means that the heart and kidneys are being put under extra strain. It is essential for your blood pressure to be checked regularly, which is why you will have it taken each time you visit the specialist or the clinic.

Having a blood pressure check

It might help if you understand what the nurse or doctor is looking for as they wrap a Velcro cuff above your elbow and pump it up so much that you feel as though your arm is going to pop. They listen to your pulse with a stethoscope and the blood pressure machine takes two measurements. One is the upper range of your blood pressure; the other is the lower. The top one is called systolic and the bottom diastolic. A 'normal' BP is something in the region of 120/80. The key figure they are checking is the diastolic. If it is raised a bit to 90 they will take note to monitor it closely, up to 100 might mean that you need treatment, and anything above that will invariably lead to you having to take medication to bring the blood pressure back down.

Treatments for raised blood pressure

There are several drugs that doctors use which have limited side effects, and this is one field where new drugs are being developed all the time. Diuretics, or water pills as they are known, can also be used. They literally help to lighten the body's load of fluids and thereby alleviate the blood pressure. You have to be careful about the dose you use, though, as diuretics can lead to dryness, dehydration and the loss of important chemicals like potassium from the body, which can result in cramps. If you are put on medication for your

97

blood pressure it is likely that you will be on it for some time. The good news is that in the majority of cases there are few if any side effects – you won't even notice you are on the pills.

Hughes syndrome

As previously mentioned, there are 'cross-over' diseases that people with lupus can have. About 30 per cent of people with lupus suffer from Hughes syndrome, or sticky blood (*see page 54*). To prevent clots – which can be potentially life threatening – those affected are given medication that makes the blood less likely to 'thicken', or coagulate. The main drugs used for this are junior aspirin, antimalarials, warfarin and heparin.

Aspirin and antimalarials

It is remarkable to think that this disease which can do so much damage can be successfully controlled by using nothing stronger than a small dose of aspirin – 75 mg a day which is a quarter of a standard aspirin tablet. As Hughes syndrome is still relatively new the body of evidence surrounding treatment for it is limited but the effectiveness of aspirin is clear. Low dose aspirin is used to help almost 100 per cent of lupus patients who have sticky blood, it is only not used in the rare cases where someone has an allergic reaction to aspirin. For instance it is known to help in pregnancy – women who have had recurrent miscarriages benefit from taking aspirin as it prevents tiny clots forming in the fine capillaries that support the baby via the placenta. Aspirin also helps with other symptoms of sticky blood; crucially it helps prevent thrombosis in the veins and arteries which can lead to strokes or heart attacks. Sometimes a patient will prove to be allergic to aspirin, in which case they might be given other medication. One widely used alternative to aspirin is called clopidogrel or Plavix.

Antimalarials are an important drug in the treatment of autoimmune diseases. They are prescribed in low doses over a long period of time and are known to be useful in preventing flares. This drug is favoured by physicians as it is mild, effective in milder cases of disease and generally has no side effects.

Warfarin

Warfarin is the standard treatment for Hughes syndrome, and in many countries it is known by the product name Coumadin. It is very effective in the control of Hughes syndrome and is much stronger than aspirin, working by altering the actual clotting system of the blood. Taken orally, it is relatively free from side effects and is used in cases where someone has had what doctors describe as a thrombotic episode, meaning that they have had a serious blood clot possibly in the limbs, lungs or brain. It is also used when someone has had a stroke.

To prevent further clotting it is crucial to get the blood-thinning end of the treatment right. The international normalisation ratio (INR) is measured, which involves looking at the thickness of a patient's blood compared with that of what you would find in normal blood. Dr Hughes states that the blood must be kept thinner by a ratio of two to three. In some people even a slight thickening of the blood will lead to symptoms like headaches or clots. You can get hold of your own blood-testing kits so that you don't have to go through the trek to hospital and the wait for results. These kits are currently rather expensive, costing in the region of £300 to £400, and you can get them from most larger chemists.

The one real side effect of warfarin to watch out for is the increased risk of bleeding. A lot of people who are on anticoagulants are fearful that they might have a serious bleed that cannot be stopped. This is unlikely as long as you work closely with your specialist. Regular tests will monitor any blood loss, and an adverse reaction will lead to a lower dose being prescribed, or to you being taken off the drug altogether.

Heparin

This is the least used anticoagulant drug for Hughes syndrome, mainly because it is administered by injection, usually just beneath the skin on the thighs or stomach. This can be uncomfortable and lead to bruising. Heparin does, however, have a number of plus points that make it a useful medication in certain circumstances. Unlike warfarin, heparin is safe to use in pregnancy – and it is important to thin the blood at this time to prevent tiny blood clots. The effects of heparin reverse quickly once it has been stopped, so it is useful for people who are about to undergo surgery, where excessive bleeding cannot be risked. It is also a fast worker: heparin will start to do its stuff within a few hours, whereas warfarin can take a number of days.

Depression

There is a variety of different drugs for depression and the general rule is that all of them can be equally effective. The trick is to realise that it might take some time to get the right drug for you tailored to the right dose. It's unfortunate that there is still a stigma attached to taking these medications because the use of them and the understanding of how they function has progressed dramatically in recent years.

Having to take antidepressants does not mean that you have lost the plot. It doesn't mean that you are weak, but simply that you have a medical problem that can be effectively treated. The fact is that if you are depressed you are likely to need antidepressants. They are not addictive like heroin, cocaine and LSD, which are drugs that act directly on the brain to replace neurotransmitters. Antidepressants act in a more indirect way to restore the natural balance of neurochemistry.

You will not be on antidepressants for the rest of your life – just long enough to sort out the depression. Exactly how long you need to take them relates to the severity of the depressive illness. The newer antidepressants are quite specific in their action and have relatively few side effects like drowsiness, dry mouth and a feeling of detachment. If for some reason, though, you cannot take the newer types, the older generation of these drugs will do the job just as well. Doctors use a broad range of antidepressants in lupus.

St John's wort

This is a herb extract from the hypericum plant and has been used for centuries to deal with low mood. Research has shown that it is effective for lupus patients who have mild depression. The thing to remember is that it can take a number of weeks for it to kick in and that might not be enough to help someone who is struggling with depression. It can be used in conjunction with other antidepressants. It is not prescribed, but can be bought in most chemists and health food shops. Evening primrose oil is another herb that is advocated for use in depression.

Tricyclic antidepressants

These have been around for half a century or more and are still widely used to treat depression and anxiety. Because they have been in common use for so long doctors know a lot about how they work and the possible side effects. They are non-addictive, and have a general impact on a person. They tend to be sedating and are likely to interact with other drugs. Tricyclic antidepressants are used in pain clinics to deal with chronic pain, but their main use is for depression involving biological symptoms. They also help to promote restful sleep. The best-known tricyclic antidepressant in non-psychiatric practice is imipramine.

Selective serotonin reuptake inhibitors (SSRIs)

These are one of the newer groups of antidepressants. They have fewer side effects than the older types because they are more specific in their action. Fluoxetine, or Prozac, falls into this group. You are less likely to get dry mouth, constipation and drowsiness if you are on these drugs than you would be if taking some other antidepressants.

Drugs for sedation

Drugs that are used for sedation, like Valium and Librium, are generally avoided these days as it is known that they are highly addictive. A doctor may, however, resort to them if a person cannot cope with alternative medication.

Sleeping tablets

Sleeping tablets are like Valium in that they have unwelcome side effects, including addiction, and should therefore only be taken for a short period of time during a crisis. If there is a longer term sleeping problem it could be due to depression, in which case antidepressants would be more appropriate.

Consultant neurologist Dr Mohammed Sharief favours the use of SSRIs because they are specific and therefore limit side effects.

I like to use SSRIs as they block certain chemicals in the brain that exacerbate the depressive mood. They have less side effects than the tricyclic drugs. I used to use Prozac but I don't any more because some patients found it unsettling, so now I use Seroxat, which is based on a natural hormone and works by specifically readjusting certain chemical levels in the brain. I avoid giving people sleeping pills for a number of reasons. Firstly, they are addictive; secondly, they can cause memory problems. What I sometimes use is a drug called Zopiclone, which is non-addictive and only works for a short period of time. It is very important to be careful what type of drug you use in lupus as you are tweaking the amount of chemicals in the brain. It is best to use a drug that acts like a magic bullet aimed at a particular target.

Dr Sharief also advocates the use of evening primrose oil.

Evening primrose oil has a calming effect. Like St John's wort it is a natural product and doesn't have many side effects. The beauty of evening primrose is that it has a lot of omega 3 and omega 6 compounds in it, so it keeps the joints supple; it is good for the skin and muscles so it is safer and has a lot of benefits.

Pain

In the majority of people who have lupus the treatments outlined above will bring down inflammation and thereby deal with pain. Many people are, however, also given specific painkillers. There are numerous options, and this is something that you should discuss with your doctor. Aspirin is recommended, but it can sometimes cause damage to the gut, nausea and (rarely) internal bleeding.

Marijuana

These days the much more relaxed legal approach to marijuana, or cannabis has resulted in some people turning to marijuana as an alternative to heavy-duty painkillers. A surprising number of people with lupus who got in touch with me about this book said that they found that smoking or eating marijuana really helped during a flare and meant they didn't have to take strong painkillers, which produced side effects like nausea, dizziness and headaches.

Annette from New Jersey in the US has been struggling with painful joints all her life. She is in her early thirties and has three young children, so she can ill afford the mornings where it takes her several hours to get out of bed because she is so stiff with joint inflammation. She was happy to share her experience of using marijuana but did not want to be identified because it is still illegal and she didn't want her friends and family to know that she was resorting to an illegal substance to help her deal with lupus.

I sometimes feel like a ninety-year-old woman because every bone, muscle and joint hurts.

The pain can be so bad that it feels as though I have been repeatedly run over by a truck. High doses of aspirin did help but then I had to stop taking so much as it was making me dizzy and nauseous. I do not want to take prescription medications. I have been afraid of them ever since my aunt became addicted to painkillers.

A few years ago I decided to try marijuana for the pain. I had read about people using it for multiple sclerosis and wondered if it might work for me. I tried it in the privacy of my own home, away from the children so they didn't know what I was doing. I found that when I smoked a marijuana cigarette the pain in my joints, muscles and bones became bearable. Having less pain meant that I could do more for the children and my mood lifted. I no longer felt so depressed about having lupus.

I have also found that my stomach didn't get so upset [as it did when she was taking aspirin] and I could eat more. I used to get panic attacks and they have gone. I found that I could relax and get on with my life. Marijuana gives me an immediate response, unlike conventional medications that take longer to have some effect. Certainly, marijuana has helped me and I intend to keep on using it to help with the pain whether it is legalised or not.

A word of warning, though. There are still a lot of unknowns when it comes to using marijuana as a painkiller. For instance, it isn't clear what potential side effects there are over long periods of time, and there have been no studies into lupus and the use of this drug. So, before you give it a try make sure you have discussed this with your doctor and perhaps others who have tried marijuana. You also need to remember that no matter how relaxed the law has become, marijuana is still illegal.

★   ★   ★

This chapter has dealt with conventional medications that are used to treat the conditions that are part of lupus. The next chapter provides ideas for complementary measures you might like to try.

Chapter 8

Complementary Measures

Lupus is not a disease to be treated lightly. It is a potential killer, and with that in mind you must think carefully before embarking on 'alternative' measures to treat it. The lupus clinic at St Thomas' Hospital often has to deal with what it calls 'the Friday admissions', where patients have stopped taking their prescribed medication on the Monday in favour of using an alternative treatment only to find that their symptoms have flared dramatically after a few days. Whatever you decide to try, do not stop taking the medication you are on without first talking to your specialist. Lupus is a tricky and complex disease, and no matter how well versed a therapist is about SLE, they will not have the same grasp of the subject as your specialist mainstream doctor.

When it comes to diet and lifestyle changes you will find that there are numerous things that people with lupus have tried that work well, and a few tell their stories later in this chapter. It is largely down to you to try things out and see what helps, as there are no hard and fast rules. If you find swimming relieves your joint pain, then do it but do not overdo it. The same applies to any exercise.

Alternative medical treatments

Most lupus specialists are reticent when it comes to recommending alternative treatments. The problem lies with the fact that there is limited research into the wide variety of products available and how effective they are in relation to lupus. So whatever you take will not necessarily have guaranteed results, and might even make your condition worse. Having said that, there is no reason not to give alternative treatments a go so long as you tread warily, do your research and check with your doctor that what you are planning will not have an adverse effect on your current treatment.

You will not be alone in looking for alternatives. The clinic at St Thomas' Hospital did a survey of its patients and found that more than 60 per cent of them had tried or were trying treatments other than those prescribed by the doctors. The team felt that as long as this did no harm then it wasn't a problem. There is in fact evidence that some products are really effective. Take glucosamine, for example. It is generally recognised in the medical speciality of rheumatology as a useful treatment for relieving inflamed joints. The negative part of this is that it is expensive to buy over the counter.

Diet and vitamins

The subject of 'diet and disease' is a massive one, and it is at the heart of a global multi-billion pound industry. This is an area in which lupus sufferers should tread carefully. If you have SLE you have to be very careful about what food supplements you decide to take. For instance, many products are designed to boost the immune system, but in lupus this is the last thing you want to do as your immune system is already running riot. You will also find that many alternative health specialists know little about lupus. You need to guard yourself against walking away from a health food shop with an armful of products and a hole in your pocket. You could find that at best the supplements are useless, and at worst they are dangerous. For instance, recent research in the US has shown that certain Chinese herbs contain steroids, so taking them on top of prednisolone could mean that you would be altering your dose without even being aware of it.

There is no specific diet recommended for lupus. Most doctors will tell you that there is no evidence that altering your diet will help. They will simply say that you must ensure you have a good balance of protein, carbohydrates and fat. Research in this area is limited, so there are no hard and fast guidelines, but clinical experience with lupus shows that there is undoubtedly a connection between worsening symptoms and certain foods. This means there are things patients can do to help themselves.

A lot of lupus patients are highly allergic, not only to insect bites but also to certain foods. For instance, it isn't uncommon to see Chinese patients whose lupus gets worse when they have eaten monosodium glutamate (MSG), a flavour enhancer used in Chinese foods. Once they stop eating foods containing MSG the aches and pains lessen.

If you see a dietician make sure they are qualified and have experience with lupus. The alternative to spending a lot of money on diet specialists is to have a go at figuring out for yourself what foods make you better or worse. Keep a detailed diary of your diet and when you have bad day track back and see what you have eaten in the past twenty-four to forty-eight hours. The potential culprits include dairy produce, wine, gluten and colouring in foods. Unfortunately there is no easy way of testing for this – the answers lie in closely monitoring your intake.

Red wine in particular appears to be a common trigger. This has nothing to do with the alcohol, though. It is thought the fermentation process could be responsible, and there is a suggestion that the sulphur content might have something to do with it. People with Hughes syndrome can also find that even the smell of white wine can bring on headaches and nausea.

There is no doubt that drinking plenty of water will help. It sounds sensible, but a lot of us don't drink enough of it and wander around unaware that we are in a mild state of dehydration (cups of coffee and tea are not good substitutes for water). If you drink two litres of water or more a day you will notice a difference. Water helps to flush out the toxins that build up in the body, especially if you are having kidney problems. Some people find that including certain herbs and vegetables – in particular garlic, parsley and onions – in their daily diet helps.

This is what Mary Baker, who has already been mentioned in Chapter 7, had to say about her diet.

Although I like a drink of alcohol I also drink two and a half litres of water a day. I used to drink half a litre overnight. I would go to bed with two or three mugs of water. I think that has been very good at flushing things out. I take so many drugs.

I believe in blood cleansing, I think it is important when you are taking so many drugs, putting lots of chemicals through your system. I must say that recently I was on water for four days and my skin hasn't looked so good for twenty years. Water flushes things through the system. I take a diuretic that makes sure it does come through the system.

You can eat things like melon to help things out; it acts as a diuretic.

The main things that I eat are garlic, parsley and onions. I eat huge quantities of those foods. I would say I eat onions five times a week, parsley goes into everything and I eat garlic five times a week. They are blood cleansers and they are really good for you. I would quickly notice if I stopped taking them – I wouldn't feel so good. I also have coriander, lemongrass and ginger.

Additionally, I think you find that as you get older there are certain things that change in your metabolism. For instance, I have been very wary of dairy foods during the last ten years. They make me feel nauseous. If you are taking tablets you really don't want to be feeling like that. I don't have milk in my tea, or butter on my toast. People's tolerance for things changes. If something makes you feel unwell, cut it out. I am a great believer in listening to your body – and remember it is yours, not the doctor's. There is only one person you have to be responsible for, and that is you.

We do know that fish oils, which contain the omega fatty acids, are good for painful joints as they have an anti-inflammatory effect, so eating oily fish like salmon and mackerel should help. Vitamin B12 and folic acid are good for anaemia, which can occur in lupus. If you are concerned about thinning bones due to steroids, taking good Vitamin D tablets or ensuring you get Vitamin D through your diet will help. Recommended sources of this vitamin include fish, butter, liver and cod liver oil, which is loaded with Vitamin D.

As previously mentioned (*see page 87*) steroids can increase your appetite and lead to weight gain. When you are on them for a prolonged time you should watch your diet carefully. It might be hard, but you should cut down on the carbohydrates and tackle the hunger pangs by having low-calorie snacks to hand. You should also increase the amount of exercise you do.

Exercise

It used to be thought that certain types of exercise could trigger a flare. We now know that this is not the case. Obviously if your joints are swollen and painful then you simply won't be able to do much weight-bearing exercise – but that doesn't mean you can't swim. The trial done at St Thomas' Hospital in London has confirmed what common sense had already told us – that exercise is good for people with lupus. The findings supported the use of appropriately prescribed graded aerobic exercise in the management of people with SLE. They found that exercise can be safely prescribed without exacerbating disease activity, and that it leads to overall improvement when compared with relaxation therapy or no intervention. The trial showed that those who did regular exercise felt much better in general, and those who kept it up beyond the study have found that their condition has improved notice-ably. One problem has been persuading patients to keep up the good work!

Elizabeth Bunn, who has lupus, exemplifies how exercise can be effective in controlling the symptoms of lupus – in particular exhaustion. After a dose of salmonella poison-ing in 1988, Elizabeth became seriously ill. Initially she experienced complications in her digestive tract alongside overwhelming exhaustion and back pain. It took years to get a diagnosis and in that time Elizabeth felt that her world was falling apart. As she often looked in good health many people around her found it hard to believe she was so unwell. The result was that she lost a lot of friends and felt isolated. The doubts of those around her made the years without a diagnosis even harder, and in the end Elizabeth moved away from her busy old life, full of pressures on her time and health, and built a new one in the West Country.

I suffered from mental fuzziness and terrible exhaustion, I was wobbly on my legs. I thought the wooden floors in my house had developed waves. I had pain in my lower back and around the back of my head and neck. I had a conviction that something was seriously wrong. I also had numbness on some areas of my body. Sometimes I would look positively blooming during a flare, other times I would go grey in the face with dark circles around my eyes. It took five years to get a diagnosis, and during that time I blamed myself for how I felt and I pushed myself harder so I could live a normal life. I saw eight consultants, then Dr Hughes was the ninth. My friends and family were despairing as all my test results were coming back relatively normal (except inflammation in the digestive tract). They began to suspect that I was neurotic – so did I.

Elizabeth wasn't imagining her fatigue and pain. Dr Hughes diagnosed lupus and the related condition Hughes syndrome (*see page 54*). Elizabeth says she's fortunate to have a swimming pool at home so she swims most days and that has helped keep symptoms at bay. She also takes regular exercise with her dog.

I have changed the way I live totally. I pace myself; if I need to rest then I do. I exercise, walking the dog or in the pool. I avoid stress as much as possible. I try to love the things I do rather than do the things I love. I paint, which makes me very happy and relaxed. I try to accept my limitations but I also accept that I will sometimes push my luck and pay the price of a flare. Swimming is so important to me. I burn up with nerve pain sometimes but the pool puts the fire out. I can dance and exercise in water but not on land as I just get muscle spasms. In the pool I can really go for it and I have got quite fit!

Physiotherapy

In lupus, mobility is an important issue. Joint pain and swelling is so bad in some people with lupus that they need help to walk, and can end up needing sticks or a wheelchair to get around. The positive news is that because the joint inflammation will generally resolve without any permanent damage, there is a good chance that you can regain some or all of the use of the affected joints. The aim is to get you back on your feet as soon as possible in conjunction with the medications that you are on to bring down swelling. A key way of achieving this is through physiotherapy. This can be limited to mild stretching, or you might be given a progressive programme of exercises. You have to bear in mind, though, that when the joints are badly inflamed you must not put too much strain on them, as this can do more harm than good and can aggravate the disease. In the light of this, physiotherapy is something that should be arranged through your doctor; take advice from your specialist. Done correctly, physiotherapy in someone who has the lupus under control can be very effective, and in many cases it can help you regain free movement.

Massage

Far from being an expensive luxury, regular massage has been shown to provide a variety of benefits for people with lupus. Most importantly, it helps to relieve stress by relaxing muscles and improving blood circulation. Specialists often recommend massage to their patients. The drawback is that you will have to foot the bill yourself, and massage sessions can be quite expensive. You will also have to choose your masseuse with care – you don't want to end up in a massage parlour that has more on offer than a soothing rub-down! The best way to ensure that you get a therapist who knows what they are doing and understands lupus is by word of mouth. Ask your medical team or lupus support groups if they have details of practitioners who are tried and tested in this field.

Positive attitude

There is no doubt that the lupus sufferers who do best are the ones who take a pragmatic view. Yes, it's a nasty, debilitating and fickle disease, but if you stand up to it then you will find a way to deal with it. Positive thinking does work, especially if you have the love and support of those around you.

Charlotte Parsley is determined to be a lawyer; in her view the lupus that has been part of her life since she was a little girl will not get in her way. She does whatever she must to push the lupus into the margins of her life. At the age of seventeen she has learned to deal with the cocktail of pills she has to swallow each day. Charlotte gets a lot of support from her family; her mother Marion has become an expert on the disease, as have the whole family. The importance of support if you are a lupus sufferer is dealt with later (*see Chapter 12*).

Charlotte first became ill when she was ten. Her doctor told her she had juvenile chronic arthritis, and she was treated for this. Six months later, after discovering a red rash on her face, she went back to the doctors, who discovered she had some kidney damage. She was sent to a rheumatologist after being ill for six months, and her mother was finally told that Charlotte had lupus. She feels being positive has helped her.

I find some aspects of lupus worse than others. For instance, I have to take loads of medication – about thirty tablets a day – and also inject myself once a day. It is annoying having to remember to take so many drugs and to take them at the right time. Wherever I am I need to remember my pills – whether it is at school or staying with a friend. I also find it irritating that I have to take so much care to keep the sun off my skin. Every day, no matter what time of year it is, I have to wear 30 SPF sunscreen, and when I'm on holiday it has to be 60 SPF sunscreen.

What is good is that my school and teachers are really understanding about lupus. I don't miss much school now because of the medications I take, so the illness rarely affects my work. I manage to do sports like tennis and swimming. I also enjoy dancing.

I know I am lucky to have had a lot of support from my family and friends. They all know and understand lupus these days and that helps a lot. I do wish more was being done to support young people with lupus in terms of support groups. In my area, Hitchin in Hertfordshire, all the groups are made up of people over thirty.

I am determined not to let lupus beat me. Once you get it under control it is more annoying than debilitating. I will not give in to it. I know that I cope pretty well with it and in the future I believe I will continue to deal with it. It will not affect my plans for the future – for example, I want a career in law and I will not let lupus get in the way of that.

Creating a recipe for coping

Lynn Marlow is a former publisher living in Norfolk. She has suffered from lupus most of her life but didn't know it until she was in her forties. She had to put up with being treated like a hypochondriac and receiving minimum help. She decided to take matters into her own hands and built her own regime for survival.

I suffered various symptoms over a number of years and can go back to the age of twelve, when I had a massive rash after sunbathing and was hospitalised. The rash became a common occurrence every summer and I thought nothing of it. I was also allergic to several types of medication and suffered from spontaneous bruising. It wasn't until my late thirties that I had 'strange' symptoms of painful joints and fatigue and this carried on until I was diagnosed at the age of forty-nine. I was diagnosed with lupus profundus, which is a variant on lupus erythematosus, after returning from living in St Lucia, where I became extremely ill and a biopsy was done on a lump on my face.

I had many and varied symptoms, but the worst was the extreme pain between my joints. or, as I now know, soft tissue. Across my chest, these pains would feel as though I was

117

having a heart attack and so painful that I could not talk. This led to my feeling extremely stressed and having panic attacks. I also suffered from extreme fatigue and constant adverse reactions to all types of medication. I was having really bad bouts of tachycardia, or fast heartbeat which had to be treated in hospital. The worst moments were when I was demented with pain and no one believed me. At one stage they put me in a psychiatric hospital for two weeks; it was the worst time of my life, as I truly believed I was losing my mind.

I have had almost every drug for lupus profundus. I proved to be extremely allergic to antimalarials. In fact, I had a total body rejection of it and my skin became blistered, swollen, withered and red. I was in hospital for almost a month and it took about six months before my skin became normal again. I now have steroids by injection every three months and this keeps the inflammation under some kind of control.

I tried several avenues of alternative medicine and was treated at the homeopathic hospital in London but became so unwell that I was unable to walk. I also tried Tibetan medicine, but that was even worse! Eating fresh vegetables and salads, restricting meat and carbohydrates, and having lots of tinned fish, such as herrings and mackerel, seems to help quite a lot. I have been able to lose over three stone in weight, and the less weight you carry around the better this is for painful joints. I walk as much as I can, even though this is still only a maximum of about ten minutes at a time, and have to take lots of rest in order to be able to get through each day.

Lynn's tips for coping with lupus include:

• Viewing each day as a 'new beginning'. Don't look back on how bad or good things were. Set small, achievable goals each day. No matter how insignificant they may seem, try to achieve them. If you don't – never mind. Tomorrow is another day. Never 'beat yourself up', because you 'can't'!

- Be selfish. Don't put yourself in the position of promising to do anything for anyone!

- Never take on any project in the distant future. Do not make dates if you can avoid them. Get your friends and family used to taking you for how you are on a day-to-day basis. Being unable to keep appointments and dates with people will only make you feel worse.

- Don't be embarrassed to lie down and rest wherever you are, and always tell people the truth when you don't feel well. You do not have to pretend.

- When you go to see your GP, make sure you do not wear any make-up and are looking like the living dead, otherwise your doctor is unlikely to believe you are unwell.

Lynn says she has come to terms with lupus, and has adjusted her life accordingly. She says she is very fortunate to be in a position to do this and to be as selfish as she needs to be because she lives on her own.

Yvonne Norton from the West Midlands in the UK is another woman who decided that the only way ahead was to fight. She first became ill back in 1975 and like other people with lupus at that time was told that she had only a short time to live – at best two years. She was having none of it. All these years on, despite having to use a wheelchair, neck-brace and wrist splints, Yvonne's indomitable spirit keeps her going.

After being admitted to hospital with complete heart

failure in 1975, Yvonne was told by the doctors that she had a 'collagen disease', but they didn't know which one. She was put on high doses of steroids for six months, which did not control her illness. After seeing Dr Hughes at Hammersmith Hospital, she was finally diagnosed with SLE. With time she also developed Sjogren's syndrome, Raynaud's phenomenon, irritable bowel syndrome, high blood pressure, lung problems and scoliosis of the spine. She uses a walking stick indoors and a wheelchair outdoors. She also needs to continually wear a neck collar and wrist splints to support her joints. Lupus and the various medications she has to take have also changed her appearance considerable over the years. Yvonne says:

Having lupus means that you do not know how you will be feeling from one day to the next. It often means that you may have to cancel arrangements for outings, etc., as you may be feeling too fatigued to make the effort to get ready and go out. You may need to rest for a few hours before you do go out and then be unable to function properly the next day. It can be difficult coping with changes in climate when the cold weather causes pain in your fingers and toes and the hot weather and sunshine bring rashes and joint pain. The good times when the symptoms are not too bad mean you can have a fun day out with the family, enjoy holidays, catch up on outstanding work or even reduce your medication for a while. This can give a great feeling of satisfaction and success.

Practical changes in my life have included having an extension built onto my home to provide a downstairs toilet and an office area as stairs are difficult. I also need to use certain aids such as special cutlery and cups. The main changes have been to my actual lifestyle. I was unable to run around with my sons for a large part of their childhood. I was, however, at home to help them with homework and to listen to them and encourage them in their interests. I had to give up paid employment, but this has meant that I have been able to establish the West Midlands Lupus Group and become involved with Lupus UK.

I do need help with housework, but I have learned over the years that there are more important things in life than having a pristine home – children will remember love and affection, not whether the furniture was polished every week. It is not possible to go away from home, whether it be overnight or on holiday, without much advance planning. I do, however, still travel abroad and attend the many lupus meetings and conferences, even though this means taking extra luggage and organising wheelchair transfers, etc. I have been unable to use public transport, but my husband Peter has been an excellent chauffeur, and ambulance personnel have been very kind over the years. I have been unable to push my grandchildren in their prams or take them to the park, but I am always there to read to them, help them with drawings and play games.

Yvonne's advice to other people with lupus is:

- Find out as much as you possibly can about lupus.
- Find a good medical consultant who really knows about lupus.
- Sort out the correct medication for your symptoms.
- Explain the illness and the effects it has upon you to your family and close friends.
- Make any changes that may be necessary to your home/lifestyle.
- **Put on a smile and get on with living!**

From sixteen-year-old Jonathan Deamer, who discusses his case later (*see page 146*), comes this strategy for coping with lupus.

I try to eat a generally healthy diet with lots of fruits and vegetables, but there's no food that I really have to avoid because of my condition. With the kidney involvement, I shouldn't have too much salt, caffeine, or alcohol, etc., but that's no problem. Some people with lupus find that certain foods, such as pork products, can trigger a flare, but this doesn't happen with me.

I find that even when I feel tired getting a bit of exercise, even if it's just a short walk, can make me feel much better. If I mope about the house all day I feel ill all day, but getting out and going for a walk blows the cobwebs away.

The only alternative medication I have tried is homeopathy, but soon after starting to take thuja extract every day I had a recurrence of my joint pains and went into a flare. I don't know if this was just coincidence, but you can't be too careful. I'm going to steer clear of homeopathy in future. Some people I have spoken to have told me that lupus patients should steer clear of alternative medicine at all costs, but others swear by it, so who knows? The thing is, many alternative medicines work on the basis of boosting the immune system, but that is the last thing you want when, as with lupus, the whole problem is an overactive immune system.

One thing I've learned is that you need to listen to your body. If you feel tired, take a break – don't push yourself too much. After a short rest you'll feel much better, and can get on with whatever you were doing. There's no point in struggling on when you're half asleep. And don't worry or beat yourself up too much when your illness means you can't do your work or you need to take a day off. I always have a tendency to feel guilty when I take a day off school because I feel like I'm skiving, but I have to tell myself 'I am actually ill. I need a day off and have no need to feel guilty!'

Also, stay positive. No matter how bad things have got for me, they have always got better. Lupus patients have enough things to deal with without getting depressed as well. Try to always look at the glass as being half full, not half empty. I don't think 'I only managed to do half a day at school today; I wish I could do a full day.' Instead I think 'Great, I did half a day at school! That's better than last week. I couldn't even get out of bed then.'

Part II

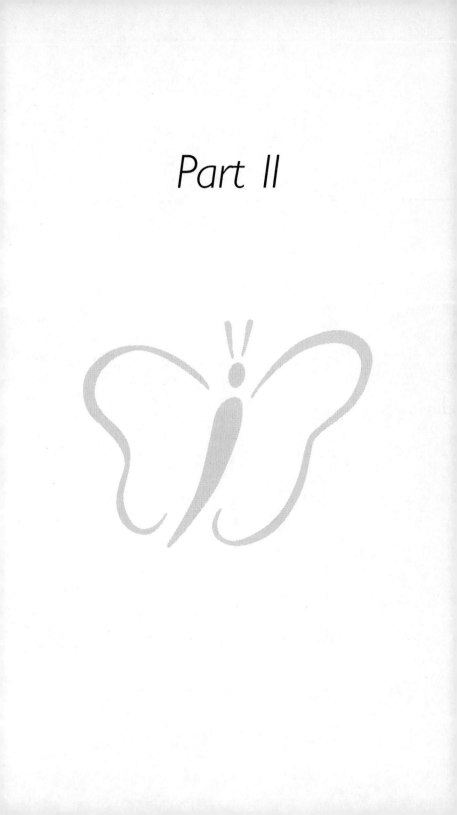

Chapter 9

Lupus and Women

It's estimated that 75 per cent of people with autoimmune diseases are women. This dramatically high figure is reflected in lupus. Nine out of ten people with lupus are female. Most new cases involve women in their early twenties, with a high percentage first becoming aware that they have the disease during or after pregnancy. No one is sure why the female of our species is the victim of choice for lupus, but it doesn't take a scientist to conclude it has something to do with hormones. As with so many things in this area of medicine, there are a lot more questions than answers. It wasn't so long ago that when you asked a doctor if hormones were involved in lupus they would have said 'no'. Now they would give you an affirmative, but would be unable to explain why.

Even worse, up until about twenty years ago the standard advice to female lupus patients was not to have children at all, and in some severe cases if a woman did get pregnant she was told to have an abortion. This guidance was based on the belief that someone with lupus had a minimal chance of carrying a child through to a successful birth, and pregnancy would put the mother at risk of having a fatal lupus flare. The story today could not be further from that grim outlook. The important thing to remember is that lupus in itself does not cause miscarriage.

Dr Hughes is fond of telling conferences about a young doctor who in the 1970s would advise SLE sufferers that on no account should they risk starting a family. He shakes his head and wonders at the naivety of this medic before revealing that it was actually himself. The pregnancy clinic at St Thomas' Hospital leads the way in this field. It has the phenomenal success rate of 85 per cent. As explained later, the news for people with lupus wanting to have children is good (*see page 131*).

The link between lupus and hormones

The close link between hormones and the immune system is known about but not well understood. As has been explained before (*see page 15*), the balance between the sexes and the number of cases is much closer in people who are pre-puberty and post-menopause – when women have less of the hormone oestrogen in their bodies – than it is in the period in between.

The majority of women have flares that link in to their menstrual cycle. In a large number of cases symptoms can be worse or reappear in the days leading up to a period. If a woman notices changes that indicate the disease is becoming more active at this time, it is possible to adjust medication to take the menstrual cycle into account. One of the things that is recognised now is that some people can keep themselves on lower doses of steroids (mini doses) for three weeks of the month and increase them in the week leading up to their period. If you fall into this category and notice that your symptoms worsen in the week before your period it is worthwhile talking to your specialist about tinkering with the dose. Don't be tempted to do this without consultation, though, as steroids are a powerful drug and it is unwise to try and go it alone (*see page 85*).

Clinical evidence over the past thirty years or more has shown that women can go into remission once their hormones 'calm down' – in other words when they have been through the menopause. How ironic that women with lupus actually have a reason to look forward to getting older!

The simplistic theory is that women's immune systems are much more complex then men's. After all, in pregnancy a woman has to carry a foetus, a foreign entity. Of course normally you would reject a foreign organism, so the immune system has to take clever action not to reject the baby. From this knowledge comes the theory that hormones alter the immune response in mild to strong ways. Certainly, laboratory tests for lupus show that if you give a mouse female hormones it gets worse, while if you give it male hormones the lupus is controlled. So at the heart of lupus are the two sex hormones oestrogen and testosterone. You can't unfortunately treat people with lupus in the way you treat mice, as the research is still in its early days, but these findings back up the belief that hormones do affect lupus.

The mechanism of hormones in relation to the immune system is complex and if you talk to leading medics in this field of research you will quickly become cross-eyed as they talk about B or T lymphocytes, cytokynes, enkephains or endorphins. If the scientists don't understand the relationship between these two crucial systems, what chance has the lay person? Dr Robert Lahita from Jersey City Hospital in New York has worked for years trying to solve this frustrating puzzle. He says the link is crucial to finding out what causes lupus, but to date we are still pretty much in the dark. He has published numerous papers on this issue and is tirelessly working on more research. He says:

> I think there are two parts to this. One is that sex hormones regulate the severity of the disease, they are not the cause; the other is that I think sex hormones or your sex predisposes you to getting an autoimmune disease. Men get lupus for sure, but men that are reproductively compromised. Men who have low levels of testosterone, men who are older, tend to have more immune problems because the immune system is not protected with testosterone. To confuse the picture even more, though, there are normal fertile virile men who get lupus – why? Well, at the moment there is no clear explanation.
>
> There is something about being a female that predisposes you to having autoimmunity. In my view it is all to do with the reproductive cycle. I do think that reproduction is the key to this. I am doing research on the ovaries in women which release the oestrogen and progesterone.

There is also research under way into the relationship between lupus and the thyroid gland. To date little is known about how the disease is connected to the thyroid, but there is clinical evidence that some women who have decreased thyroid function after the menopause tend to be more likely to get late-onset lupus, although this isn't a severe form of the disease. A large percentage of these women also reported that they had problems with low thyroid output in earlier life. Frustratingly, this information has not yet been collated, so there are no clear answers as to what the connection is beyond the fact that it obviously has to do with hormonal activity.

Can I have a baby?

If you have read some of the older books about SLE you will have ended up feeling pretty depressed and convinced that it is tricky or even impossible to have a baby if you suffer from lupus. Take heart – the clear message is 'Do not despair' and the impression you were given is false. Contrary to what has been written in the past, lupus alone does not increase the risk of miscarriage. It is the presence of Hughes' syndrome (*see page 54*) that is the critical factor in these situations. The chances of you having a healthy baby are as good as those of a non-lupus sufferer if your disease is being controlled and you take certain precautions. When you have a chronic illness and you want to have a baby you do have to be aware of the state of your health – the better you are the greater chance you have of carrying to full term. The general advice is:

• Do not try for a baby during a flare or when you are recovering from one.

• Wait for six to nine months after a flare before getting pregnant.

• Let your medical team know that you want to start a family.

• If you are already pregnant and the lupus is active remember that there are effective treatments to help you through – for instance, increasing the dose of steroids should bring the lupus under control and protect the pregnancy.

- Prepare your body for pregnancy; when you are well enough do some gentle exercise, watch your diet – cut down on carbohydrates, salt and alcohol, and ensure that you get enough sleep.

- Be aware that in some severe cases of lupus, periods can become irregular or stop altogether – this does not mean that you cannot have a baby but you will have to talk the problem through with your doctor.

Although lupus in itself doesn't cause miscarriage it can make you unwell during a pregnancy. There can be flares in the second and third trimesters but these are mostly mild. The main problems occur post-partum – just after the baby is born. The first few months after delivery – known as the puerperium – are a high-risk time as a large percentage of women with lupus have a flare at this stage. Because of this they are monitored very closely, and early symptoms need to be treated quickly. It isn't uncommon for women who did not even know they had lupus to develop the first signs of the disease in the few days after childbirth. Once again, the reason for this is hormones and the dramatic changes that women go through at this time.

Hughes syndrome and pregnancy

Things become more complicated if you have lupus and Hughes syndrome (*see page 54*). This condition, which is found in a third of people with lupus, makes the blood more inclined to clot. It can have a profound effect on pregnancy. If you have lupus it is likely that you will have had a test for antiphospholipid antibodies (*see page 69*), which will be present in your blood if you have this condition. It will be up to the specialist who is treating you to determine if there are clinical signs of the syndrome and decide if treatment is needed.

If you are unsure whether you have been tested or not, ask your doctor – it is crucial that you know whether or not you have Hughes syndrome if you are planning to become pregnant. As the blood becomes more viscous in those who have this condition, the chances of the fine capillaries in the placenta clotting are high and this can limit or prevent the blood supply to the foetus. This leads to placental insufficiency, which means the placenta can't do its job properly. If this is untreated, the pregnancy will be jeopardised.

One in five recurrent miscarriages are due to Hughes syndrome, not to lupus per se. The condition can also make getting pregnant in the first place difficult. Infertility clinics are waking up to the possibility that some women who were thought to be infertile actually had problems getting pregnant because they had this syndrome – their blood was too thick. Relatively simple treatment to thin the blood can make a dramatic difference. A high percentage of women who get the right medication go on to have successful pregnancies even when they have a long history of miscarrying.

The key is to work with your doctors. They will want to monitor you closely during pregnancy and the outcome is more likely to be good if you plan things carefully before you get pregnant. Having said that, some women don't know they have Hughes syndrome until they are having a baby as it can be present without showing any symptoms before pregnancy. Awareness of Hughes syndrome is even more limited than that of lupus. It is a relatively new disease so it is common for doctors not to have heard of it, and to have had no experience in dealing with it. A leading obstetrician says that the identification of Hughes syndrome is the biggest advance in gynaecology in recent years. If you suspect you may have this condition as well as lupus and you are having problems getting pregnant or have suffered one or more miscarriage, insist on being tested for it.

Angela Foster knew she had lupus when she became pregnant with her first child, Freddie. Although the pregnancy wasn't planned Angela, a systems engineer from Salisbury in the United Kingdom, was delighted. There was no problem conceiving and she knew her condition was mild. The diagnosis of SLE meant she was kept under the watchful eye of her specialist team. Other than a lupus skin rash on her legs and some joint pain she was relatively well. Her second pregnancy the following year also went well – baby Henry arrived in October 2000. It was a different story during Angela's third pregnancy in 2002.

> This time things didn't go so well. I had a bad flare and was off work for four months. They thought I had a virus but then I had a TIA (mini-stroke); this affected my brain and it was very scary. I went on to develop joint pains and lethargy. There was one particular occasion when I was reading a newspaper and I just couldn't comprehend the words. I tried to spell them and they still didn't make any sense. I rested for a while and tried again, and this time I could get the meaning of the words but not whole sentences. My brain wouldn't work. I tried to tell my husband what was wrong but I couldn't.
>
> It passed after a while and I just put it down to my hormones being all over the place. It was when I told my doctor about these odd symptoms that I realised something had happened to my brain function. At that point I was scared because I didn't know what was going on. I was tested for Hughes syndrome and they found the antibodies. After that I began injecting myself with Fragmin to thin the

blood. Once Mary was born I went on to Warfarin. I also take prednisolone, thyroxine and Plaquenil.

I know I am lucky to have had my three children. Other people with Hughes syndrome have had problems with conceiving and miscarriage.

Risks to the baby

The majority of medications that women take for lupus do not have an adverse effect in pregnancy, although the immunosuppressive drug methotrexate must not be used in pregnancy as it can affect the foetus. Steroids, antimalarials and even immunosuppressives like azathioprine have been shown in tests not to pose a threat to the unborn child. The alternative to stopping the drugs might be a major flare during pregnancy, which would bring with it a whole range of risks to both mother and baby. Although the drugs can be strong, the evidence is that most pose low risks. Once again it is crucial to work closely with the specialists, who will have a clear view on what medications you can safely take during a pregnancy.

An understandably common question is 'Will the baby be affected by lupus, or be born with it?' The answer is that babies are not more likely to be born with congenital abnormalities. There are, however, some risks that you should be aware of and must weigh up if you are planning a pregnancy.

With the genetic component there is a risk that a child will go on to have the disease, but this is not a strong enough factor to counsel against starting a family. The risk is 1 per cent or less – which is only marginally greater than that of children born to people who don't have lupus.

The anti-Ro antibody

More serious is the presence of a particular antibody that can have an adverse effect on a baby. A woman's blood will be tested for the anti-Ro antibody, which is found in about a quarter of women who have lupus. It is linked to Sjogren's syndrome (*see page 58*), but is also a marker for milder lupus. In very rare cases, about one in 1,000, this antibody can pass from the mother's bloodstream into the tissue of the baby's heart and lead to congenital heart block. This means that the heartbeat is slow; the pulse is roughly forty beats a minute. For the infant, the condition is potentially serious. If untreated, it can affect the normal growth and development of a child's heart, so that a cardiac pacemaker may need to be inserted to return things to normal.

Neo-natal lupus

Another potential complication is neo-natal lupus. This is where a baby develops a lupus-like rash within the first few weeks of life. This is linked to the mother's antibodies being passed in utero to the baby across the placenta. It causes an inflammation of the skin that mimics the adult version. The cutaneous rashes can look frightening and will be a terrible worry for parents, but the condition is temporary and will usually pass by the time the child is six months old, when the antibody has been naturally flushed from the bloodstream. Neo-natal lupus does not involve internal organs – only the skin.

What about breastfeeding?

As for breastfeeding, there is no problem in the majority of cases. A mother with lupus should be able to feed her child naturally despite being on a number of standard medications. Steroids, for instance, do not pass to the baby in the milk. There are, however, other drugs that might be toxic and that is why each case is assessed on an individual basis. Once again it comes down to working closely with your medical team.

Against the odds

Cheryl Marcus, the founder of Lupus UK (*see* Resources, *page 211*) has had two sons, despite having lupus for thirty years. As she struggled in the early days of her illness Cheryl decided to follow the advice of one specialist and try for a child as soon as she could. This was before her first encounter with Dr Hughes in the early 1970s and Cheryl was on hefty doses of steroids. Remarkably, during her pregnancy the symptoms calmed down and Cheryl actually felt a lot better, but the reprieve was only temporary.

After Daniel's birth the illness returned with a vengeance. During the birth I felt terribly ill – my joints were very painful. Shortly after Daniel was born I was referred to a rheumatology specialist. I was put on very high doses of steroids (100 mg per day to start with) and it was felt that larger and larger doses of this drug were my only hope of staying alive. It was obvious that the doctors did not know what to do, which made matters worse.

In fact, Cheryl became something of a medical exhibit as her condition was so severe.

I was wheeled into lecture rooms and young junior doctors were asked to find a diagnosis. I felt like a freak and due to the steroid treatment I lost all my hair and my weight ballooned from eight and a half stone to thirteen. Within a couple of months I could not walk, and felt extremely depressed and tearful. My parents and Martin, my husband, all felt so frustrated that they were unable to do anything to help me. Meanwhile having such a poor circulation caused me to have severe ulcerations on my hands and feet. My whole body hurt. And all the while our baby, Daniel, was going to and fro, being looked after by my mother and husband. After seven months the decision was made that this was unfair on him, and also that it was too hard for my parents and Martin to run two homes. It was decided that my parents would sell their home, Martin would sell ours, and we would find a large house that could be turned into two flats

A lot of this time I was in hospital, allowed home only for an occasional weekend. After eight months it was decided that I could be nursed at home. A nurse came in every day to clean me and change the dressings on the ulcers. I was in a wheelchair and needed continual help.

After a couple of months at home I suffered a convulsion. This caused me to suffer a fractured spine and I had to wear a brace from under my arms down to my hips. This was very heavy but it did reduce the pain and allowed the fractures to heal gradually.

When I saw Dr Hughes at the Hammersmith Hospital things changed completely. He was keen to work with a patient who was so ill and presented a challenge to his new knowledge. I will never forget that he told me that not only would I live, but also I would walk again, my hair would grow back and I would lose the weight. Dr Hughes gradually reduced the steroids and introduced different and sometimes experimental treatments. He continually monitored my body's reaction to the new drugs that I had been prescribed, such as immunosuppressive drugs as well as antimalarial drugs. I was also given intense physiotherapy to help me walk properly again. After eleven months spent mainly in Hammersmith Hospital I returned home. I continued to improve and was able to envisage a great future for us.

When I found I was pregnant again I had to agree to stay in hospital until the birth. I was allowed home one day a week, which was a great help to Daniel and all the family, as the journey to Hammersmith Hospital was a long one for them to undertake.

Seven months into the pregnancy it was decided that I should have an immediate Caesarean birth as the baby had stopped developing. I gave birth to a tiny two and a half pound baby son, Jonathan. His initial months in neo-natal care were turbulent for him – and us – but we were ecstatic to eventually have him home when he was eleven weeks old.

Nowadays there are special lupus pregnancy clinics to deal with cases like mine, and new treatments have revolutionised the outlook for a safe and full-term pregnancy; in fact, there are very rarely problems if people follow the clinic's advice.

Cheryl's story shows that even in the toughest cases of lupus, having a family is possible.

Oestrogen hormone treatments

You may be considering the pill (which contains oestrogen) as a contraceptive measure, or oestrogen replacement therapy, and here is some information on both. Bear in mind, however, that if you have lupus and suffer from headaches, thrombosis or high blood pressure, or have a diagnosis of Hughes syndrome, you will be strongly advised to avoid all medications that contain oestrogen.

Contraception

In light of the role hormones play in lupus it is important to take care when it comes to planning your
contraception. High–dose oestrogen pills are not recommended. You also need to avoid the combined pill that
has oestrogen in it. In some mild cases of lupus the mini-
pill can be used, but with caution – start on a 'trial and
error' basis. If symptoms start to appear you should have
a rethink about what you are taking. At the first sign of
an adverse reaction you should go back to your doctor
and try something else.

The progesterone-only pill is considered safe, and is
available either from your doctor or from your family
planning clinic – but you must remember to take it at
the same time each day. There are some side effects.
It may cause vomiting or severe diarrhoea. If you get your
contraception from a family planning clinic you must
make it clear to the person you are seeing there that you
have lupus. It is possible that they will feel unable to deal
with the disease and will want you to see your specialist.

Caution is also advised if you are considering a contraceptive implant that contains oestrogen. With oestrogen you
get an initial high dose that gradually wears off over a period
of weeks. Clinical evidence of patients using this method of
contraception is that it can make you ill and that lupus symptoms may be tickled up when the implant is first put in. The
advice is therefore to avoid this form of contraception.

Contraceptive methods that are considered safe include
the intrauterine contraceptive device (IUCD/IUD), or coil,
in particular the progesterone coil – although you have to
watch out for any pelvic inflammation. Other methods that
are recommended are male and female condoms and the
diaphragm, also known as the cap.

If you have lupus it is important to make sure you think through your contraception options carefully, and talk them through with your specialist to ensure you find a method that suits you.

Hormone replacement therapy (HRT)

In light of the evidence that certain hormones appear to trigger lupus, you might find it surprising that HRT is considered relatively safe for lupus sufferers. This is because it contains low doses of oestrogen. About ten years ago the Rayne Institute at St Thomas' Hospital published a survey that looked at HRT in patients at the hospital's lupus clinic. The results showed that it was well tolerated and did not produce flares in the majority of patients, who were found to have the same degree of improvement or otherwise on HRT as the general population. As in the case of all medications, it is wise to talk this through with your doctor.

Chapter 10

Other Groups Affected by Lupus

This chapter discusses how lupus affects three other important groups of people: children, men and specific populations of African and Asian origin.

Children

Lupus is seen in all age groups, from newborn babies onwards. At the moment the condition is regarded as being rare in children under the age of twelve or pre-puberty, but as with so many aspects of lupus, the picture is constantly changing. The number of young people with the disease is increasing, although it is hard to say whether this is because it is actually becoming more prevalent or simply because doctors are better informed and are therefore beginning to consider it more often as a diagnosis in the under sixteens. It is probably a combination of both.

It is quite common for doctors to take the medical history of adult lupus patients and find that they had certain symptoms as children that could have been early signs of the disease. Joint inflammation in the young is often diagnosed as 'growing pains'. This is a vague condition that is not regarded as medically significant and is often treated with mild painkillers or nothing at all on the basis that a child will grow out of it. The clinical evidence is that many people with lupus were told they had growing pains as children, but no one thought any more about it until they developed other symptoms years later.

Lupus and glandular fever

Many adults with lupus were told that they had glandular fever, or mononucleosis, as children or teenagers. This is an acute infection caused by the Epstein-Barr virus (EBV). It is one of the most common human viruses. In the majority of people it produces no symptoms. In some, however, particularly teenagers, it can trigger a vigorous immune reaction and make them unwell for weeks, months or in rare cases years. There is no one conclusive test for EBV and that means it can be wrongly diagnosed. The persistent and recurring swollen glands, high temperature, sore throat and flu-like symptoms might actually be lupus. Research has also been done into whether there is a link between EBV and lupus.

A 1997 study by scientists from the Oklahoma Medical Research Foundation in the US looked at children and young adults with lupus. It revealed that 99 per cent of the lupus patients tested had the EBV virus, while of the non-lupus control group only 70 per cent had it. The conclusion was that there could be a connection.

When the work was published, the headlines declared that the EBV could be the cause of lupus, but many scientists dispute this. More research is under way into the possible connection and it's frustrating that a so-called 'breakthrough' is more like a sideways step. One thing that the report did do, though, was to establish a link of some kind, and it supports the view that people with lupus are highly susceptible to the EBV. It could be possible that having the virus sets the stage for lupus later in life. Time and more research will help give some context to these findings – for instance, it might be useful to develop a vaccine against the EBV for those children who are considered to be at risk from lupus, such as those who have relatives with lupus or who have early lupus-like symptoms.

Living with lupus as a child

Having lupus at any age is a lonely business, but it is perhaps hardest on the young. Children and teenagers with this condition have to deal with the same problems as those faced by adults, as well as their own particular issues. Being sick with something that no one has heard of or can see isn't 'cool'. Missing long periods of school is tough, and not being able to do all the things their friends are doing inevitably alienates the child. Because lupus isn't particularly well known it is likely that an affected child's school will not have come across the disease before. It might be an uphill struggle to make staff understand about the long periods of absence, missed homework or the child falling asleep in lessons due to chronic fatigue. All this can be misinterpreted if teachers don't realise it is part of the disease.

The drugs a child has to take can make them put on weight, or the disease can mark their skin. Joint inflammation can make it difficult for a young person to walk or run properly, so they become less active at a time in their lives when they generally want to take part in sports activities. In these image-conscious days the pressure to look a certain way is great, so embarrassing physical changes can be devastating – even though they are invariably temporary.

Most of the support networks that exist are designed for people in their twenties onwards. There is a great need for children who are affected by lupus to be able to speak to others who are in the same boat. While working on this book I spoke to numerous children with lupus and they were desperate to link up with other young people who had the same condition. Nothing helps you feel less like an alien than meeting people who are like you. There are several websites that can help young people (*see page 211*), but the fact remains that there is still no real support network targeted at this age group.

Another factor that needs to be taken into account is the lack of awareness among young people. Recent research in the US has shown that the highest level of ignorance about lupus was among the under eighteens, yet this is the age where knowledge and early diagnosis can help people come to terms with lupus and set a pattern for a normal life.

Sixteen-year-old Jonathan Deamer, who has already been mentioned earlier (*see page 121*), has been sick with lupus since he was eight. The fear and uncertainty of being so unwell at such a tender age left a mark both on Jonathan and on his family. His parents Gill and Kevin and his younger brother Matthew found that their lives were also affected by lupus, and they had to cope with years of not knowing what was wrong and watch help-lessly as Jonathan's condition deteriorated. Jonathan, who lives in Farnborough in Hampshire, England, had never been a sickly child, and his early symptoms of joint pains and headaches didn't worry his doctor unduly. It was only when he began to pass red urine that he was admitted to hospital. Jonathan wants to be a writer and the follow-ing is his own account of how lupus has affected him and his loved ones.

Until the age of eight I had been completely healthy, but then I started becoming more and more more unwell. For months I was generally run down and tired and missed lots of school. I found it completely impossible to get up in the morning, and seemed to have a permanent cough or cold. We went back and forth to the doctor's more times than I care to remember, only to be given a course of antibiotics each time, or something equally useless. I also developed a terrible rash all over my chest and back, which at the time was dismissed as 'urticaria', or hives. It is apparently quite common and nothing to worry about, but looking back now I realise that this was actually one of my first signs of lupus. Things continued like this for a while, and then I started passing blood in my urine. We went to the doctor's again, but even with a urine sample that was the colour of red wine, I was still sent away and told there was nothing wrong with me.

One Saturday morning I woke up feeling worse than ever, and my dad took me to the emergency clinic and demanded to see someone straight away. We saw a different doctor from my usual one, and I was then admitted to our local hospital, Frimley Park. This was in March 1996. All they could tell was that I had 'some kind of kidney problem'.

I found the whole thing very frightening. I was just nine years old, and on top of the fact that I was being told I had a serious illness was the trauma of being admitted to hospital. I was surrounded by doctors and nurses, all asking me questions. The doctors didn't know what was wrong with me, so what was I meant to think? Was I going to die? It sounds like a stupid thing to say, but I was very young and didn't understand what was going on. I had a cannula – a plastic tube – connected to my arm so the doctors could take blood easily, and even this simple thing seemed a big trauma at the time – now it would be nothing.

After a night at Frimley Park, I was sent to Guy's Hospital in London, where I had hundreds of blood tests and a kidney biopsy. These showed that I had acute inflammation of the glomerulus – which are the filtering units in the kidneys. They believed this was caused by my immune system attacking my kidneys, but there was no firm diagnosis. There were a whole host of things they believed it might be, but nothing conclusive, so for the moment the doctors went with the diagnosis of Henoch-Schonlein purpura nephritis – which means an inflammation of the small capillaries in the kidneys causing a leakage of blood. This seemed to be the only thing that matched my symptoms at the time.

I started taking prednisolone steroids, which did the trick, and within a few days I stopped passing blood in my urine and felt much better all around. For the next couple of months I was up and down a bit, finding the right dose and adjusting to all the medication, but all in all I felt much better than I had done for the last year.

For the next few years I was treated as an outpatient at Guy's Hospital, and for the most part I was completely well, but every year whenever we tried to reduce my dose of steroids to below 10 mg a day, the kidney problem became active again. Apart from taking my tablets every day, and occasionally checking my urine for blood, I could just lead a normal life. I even managed to play rugby regularly. At this stage we had never even heard of lupus.

When I was thirteen, however, I began getting some strange symptoms. I had seemingly permanent headaches. I sometimes found it hard to breathe, and I started getting heart palpitations. The doctors were very interested in all these things – because I had never had a firm diagnosis, they began to think 'Could these things be connected?' I had

147

every test under to sun – brain scans, twenty-four-hour heart
and blood pressure monitors, breathing tests, but all proved
inconclusive. They even tested for lupus and sent blood
samples to different labs all over the country, but all the tests
came back negative. We thought nothing of it at the time,
but later we realised the significance of these symptoms. For
the moment, however, they all went away and I continued
living a mostly healthy life.

A year later my left wrist was hurting a bit. After a week,
the pain had spread to my shoulder. Finally, when I tried to
get out of bed a few days later, I found I was unable to
walk. Now my knees and ankles didn't just ache a bit, they
really hurt. My fingers, wrists, elbows – basically every joint in
my body was really painful. I then stayed off school for the
next four weeks.

I slept all day, and couldn't sleep at night because of
the pain, even though I was incredibly tired, and I got really
bad mouth ulcers. I stopped eating, and my weight went
down to nine stone – not healthy for a fourteen-year-old,
almost six-foot-tall rugby player. I went back and forth to
the doctors only to be told 'It might be flu. Then again, it
could be glandular fever. Either way, bed rest will do the
trick' and I was given a prescription for painkillers. At this
point we never thought it could be connected to my other
problems.

Then one of the blood tests, which I'd had done hundreds
of times before, suddenly started giving a different reading. An
intravenous steroid drip worked straight away – the next
morning I got up and went out in search of the nearest
McDonalds breakfast. This was a great relief, after a month
of having no appetite and being unable to walk unsupported.
My kidney doctor now told us he believed it could be a thing
called lupus. After another couple of days of intravenous
steroids, I felt completely well again, and went back to school

a week later. I was then referred to the lupus specialist at St Thomas' Hospital, Dr Graham Hughes.

The doctor at the clinic examined me and did various tests, including the Shirmer's dry eye test, which I had never had done before. This was because my mother has Sjogren's syndrome, the immune condition that causes dry eyes, nose and mouth, and is connected with lupus.

Finally – after seven years – it was confirmed that I had lupus. I started a new medicine called CellCept, also known as mycophenolate. This is a pioneering new 'wonder drug', which suppresses the immune system like steroids do, but without all the side effects. At first, I felt worse – in fact now I couldn't even go to school. After being off school for about another three weeks and missing all my mock exams, the stomach pains and nausea went away as my body got used to the new tablets. I began to find getting up in the morning easier, and my joints got a little less painful each day. I looked forward to slowly coming off the steroids.

I've been lucky in that I've had very supportive family, friends and teachers. My parents do everything they can to look after me, and they have a very positive outlook, which helps me cope. My friends always ask me how I am, and look out for me, and they understand if I have to let them down because I'm unwell. My teachers at school are all aware of my illness, and they don't pressure me too much when I can't always hand in homework on time or revise for a test. The doctors at the kidney unit have also been wonderful, and I always know I could contact them any time. They have done their best to help me, even outside of their area of expertise, when I was having heart or lung problems.

I think the future looks pretty good. I hope my CellCept continues to work and I can get off the prednisolone completely by next summer sometime. My doctors say that *by then, all being well, I should be able to come off even the CellCept and take some other drug to just keep the lupus at bay. I don't know if by then I will still have permanent day-to-day tiredness and aching joints, but I'm learning to adapt my lifestyle, so I'll be able to deal with that.*

Although it is hard to come to terms with having an illness like lupus, there is no doubt that those who do best are the patients who get on with their lives. These are people who treat the condition like an unwelcome guest that they put up with but keep firmly in its place. You have to learn to control the lupus and not the other way around. A positive outlook is of key importance (*see page 115*). Examples of the greatest courage come from young people who face a lifetime's struggle against lupus with pragmatism and tenacity.

Men get it too

Inevitably the question arises – if lupus is related to the female hormone, oestrogen, then why does it also affect males who are loaded with testosterone? To date there is no answer to this. Doctors are still groping around in the dark, trying to understand why this is the case. Certainly the figures for the incidence of lupus show dramatic changes in the male/female ratio in different age groups. Obviously it has to do with hormone levels, but there is no conclusive research to explain the exact reason for it.

Men with lupus can have an especially tough time. Lupus is seen as a 'woman's disease', with only 10 per cent of people suffering from it being male. The knock-on effect is that men who have it can feel stigmatised and isolated.

When they attend clinics they can find themselves being the lone male patient in a waiting area packed with women and children. Support groups are often geared up for women, and even chat rooms on the Internet have few male participants. This creates another raft of difficulties to cope with on top of the illness.

One of the most important things for men with lupus to know is that having this condition does not make you less masculine. Men with this condition have normal sperm counts and are just as capable of fathering children as men who don't have lupus. Their characteristics – hair, voice, muscles and so on – are what you would expect in a sample of the wider male population.

Essentially the disease is the same in men as in women, although it does appear to be more aggressive. All the symptoms described in women – other than those to do with the menstrual cycle and pregnancy – are seen in men. The treatment is the same for men as for women. As is the case with women, lupus may be seen in a man's family history, or it can be brought on by the triggers mentioned in Chapter 1 (*see pages 17–25*). Clinics see a higher ratio of men with lupus as a result of certain drugs, antibiotics in particular. It is thought that this is because the medications that can cause drug-induced lupus are used more often in men than in women.

Studies show that men with lupus do worse than women, and that their condition is more active, and proves to be more difficult to treat. The reasons for this aren't known. You would expect men's testosterone levels to protect them against this severity of the disease. Whether it's because these men have lower testosterone levels than other men isn't known. Another factor is that some GPs may not think of lupus as a man's disease. As a result, male sufferers may be ill for some time before getting a diagnosis and treatment

– they may be seen by specialists at a much later stage of the disease than women generally are.

An indication of how ferocious lupus can be comes with the story of Aneal Advani. He was a young man with a bright future. In his twenties he had built up a brilliant career with a major investment bank in the City of London. Aneal had a large salary and good looks, and was bursting with energy. There was little doubt among his peers that he would go far. But life had other plans for him.

When Aneal was twenty-seven years old he developed flu-like symptoms, and his condition rapidly deteriorated. He had a high fever, fatigue and joint problems. He became so ill that he had to be admitted to hospital. Over a period of weeks he became more and more unwell. The fever did not abate and movement became difficult because of joint inflammation. He also began to develop a butterfly rash across the cheeks of his face and the bridge of his nose. At the time he did not realise how significant this was. His symptoms puzzled doctors, and for over twenty months they carried out endless tests without finding anything conclusive. They gave a diagnosis of possible tuberculosis. It was a chance encounter with a locum doctor that finally pinned down what was really wrong with Aneal.

I first became ill in March 1998, with symptoms of fever, extreme fatigue, sweats and abdominal pain. My fever kept going higher and before I knew it I was in hospital. While there I developed more symptoms, such as joint pains, swollen joints and swollen glands. I then went on to develop what I know now as a butterfly rash. For about twenty months I was used as a pincushion and tested for just about everything. They thought that I was suffering from TB, but they didn't really have a clue what was wrong. I had seen many doctors over that period of time but it was only pure luck that led me to the answer.

My usual doctors were away so I saw another specialist. He immediately spotted the symptoms of lupus and had me tested. I had never even heard of the disease before this. The results were positive and I was sent to see Dr Hughes, the leading British doctor in this field. It turned out that I also had Hughes syndrome, which makes the blood more likely to clot. Unfortunately, this progress after twenty months of being so ill came too late to stop me from having a major stroke. I don't know if it was caused by the lupus or the Hughes syndrome, but it did permanent damage. The result is that I have problems with memory and thought processes. I have not been able to work since then. The impact on my life could not have been more profound.

Aneal's lupus is particularly aggressive. Getting a diagnosis undoubtedly saved his life, but the disease has been and continues to be difficult to treat. Aneal has found himself at death's door on a number of occasions, and each time huge doses of medication were needed to bring the flare under control. He never knows from one day to the next how he will be, and that uncertainty puts enormous pressure on himself, his wife Jana and the rest of his family.

The most difficult symptoms to live with are the ones that affect my 'normal' activities. My joint pains and stiffness prevent me from doing things that I enjoy. For the last few months my joints have tended to swell and fill up with fluid if I do too much. Unless the pain gets really bad I seem to be able to cope with it better each day. I think this is because I have grown accustomed to having it there all the time. When the disease starts to flare up, Jana and

I both recognise the signals and race off to the lupus unit, where these days they immediately give me a large dose of intravenous steroids. During these times I often look quite well. These 'signals' have to be addressed immediately or the flare gets uncontrollable and I end up in hospital.

On the three occasions that I have had major flares I have nearly died. The most recent occasion was the most frightening as I was actually aware of everything and knew that there was nothing that we could do about it. Nowadays, things have settled and I have to deal with the relatively minor problems of the extreme fatigue and pain. I can be fine one minute and then all of a sudden I've passed out and wake up a couple of hours later not knowing what happened. The pain is dealt with using painkillers when it is bad, but otherwise I just grin and bear it. I have cerebral lupus and have had some after effects from the flares. Each day is different, though, and one never knows what the next day is going to be like.

I have other diseases that are related to the autoimmune family. One of them is Hughes syndrome and the other is myositis. Surprisingly, I seem to be the only one in my family who has any of these autoimmune problems. Of course I am pleased that no one else in my family has them but it raises the question as to why I got them. It is made even harder by the fact that lupus is more common in women so I am definitely considered to be strange. When I attend meetings to do with lupus I am often surrounded by women.

I think that lupus is a mental disease as well as a physical one. You have to be strong mentally or it will drag you down to the lowest point in your life. Being positive and having people around you who are positive yet understanding is very important.

Coping with lupus has been and continues to be very difficult. Looking well on the outside but feeling awful on the *inside, the constant pain, people's ignorance and the constant uncertainty of life will always be difficult to deal with. I have to stress that anything I say is referring to my case only, as it is well known that lupus affects people differently. Currently, my medication can keep the disease under control and providing we are extremely vigilant I hope to hang on until they find a solution.*

As I have mentioned earlier in this book (*see page 15*), the ratio of men affected by lupus is much higher in children and people over fifty-five. The disease can make an unwelcome appearance in those who have been perfectly healthy all their lives. Becoming ill can change how people behave, as can the condition itself or the medications used to treat it. Certainly there is growing evidence that the vast majority of people with lupus suffer from some form of neurological involvement. Often it is hard to differentiate what the trigger is – after all, who wouldn't feel down if they had a long-term illness?

Brian Hayes from Bradford in West Yorkshire, England, firmly believes that it was the immunosuppressive drug methotrexate that turned him into a Jekyll and Hyde character. He went from Mr Nice to Mr Nasty almost overnight. From a medical viewpoint this is more likely to have been brought on by the lupus; methotrexate is not known to cause psychotic problems, whereas it is a recognised symptom of SLE. Brian was undiagnosed for three years, which would have given the lupus plenty of time to affect his behaviour.

Brian had been a craftsman all his life. He left school young to train as a stonemason. Specialising in restoration, he worked at his trade for forty-six years. He didn't drink or smoke and kept fit, and in all those years had never missed a day of work through illness.

I was super-fit – I had to be as the work was very physically demanding. I was always careful about my health so it was a shock when I started to have joint problems in my hands when I was fifty-nine. I thought it had something to do with the new equipment I had been using – in order to compete stonemasons switched to using pneumatic hammers that had come in from the Italian marble quarries. Obviously the vibration of the equipment had an effect on your hands. I continued to work as best I could but it was painful as my hands were so bad. My fingers were swollen and I was finding that I had become tired all the time. I saw my doctor, who got some tests done and it was decided that I had rheumatoid arthritis. The doctor told me that I had to retire as I was no longer well enough to do such strenuous work. It was a terrible wrench.

As time went by the treatments I was getting for the arthritis didn't seem to be helping. The worst thing for me was how my character changed after I was put on methotrexate. I had just been diagnosed with lupus and none of us really understood what that was. I began to act strangely. I got quite nasty. Nothing was right for me. I was always bad tempered and had no time or patience for anyone or anything. I wouldn't sit down, couldn't concentrate – I wasn't able to read or watch TV for long. I wasn't fit to live with. It was most distressing as I had always been a gentle person, not at all like this. I developed migraine, my hair fell out and the skin on the soles of my feet started coming off. I was also really tired – I would sleep all day and night and wake up exhausted. All of this was so unlike me. I was on the methotrexate for six months, and in the end I refused to take it any more. Once I stopped and took other medication my mood gradually improved. I am fairly sure it was the methotrexate, although I still have problems with concentration.

Brian goes on to say:

> I recommend that people contact support groups. This is where they will find up-to-date information and they can talk to other people with this disease. Unless you have it you cannot begin to understand what it's like.

One of the keys to coping with lupus, whether you are male or female, is to follow Brian's example and find others like yourself. You might discover that it helps to talk about your own experiences as well as listen to others about theirs. If you have access to the Internet you will find a vast amount of information floating around on the web. When I typed in 'lupus' on one search engine I got more than a million results. It is hard to know what percentage of these are useful, but even if was only 1 per cent, that would still give you 10,000 leads to follow.

Remember not to believe all you read, and be cautious about chatting to other people with lupus who have learned so much about the disease that they are keen to offer you medical advice. With this condition more than most it takes a trained medical expert to get it right. Having said that there are plenty of sites that portray people's stories and tell how they coped.

Brett Borowski works mostly in computer programming. Brett, who lives in Princeton, New Jersey, in the United States, with his wife and four-year-old daughter, has taken a pragmatic approach to his lupus by sharing his story on the Internet. Brett has had years on a medical rollercoaster, struggling from one crisis to the next. He has suffered repeated aggressive lupus flares, and episodes of mania that were side effects from high doses of medication. Throughout this he has managed to keep a detailed diary of what he and his family have gone through. He publishes it on his own website. It is a work in progress and gives an excellent portrayal of one man's fight against lupus.

Brett shares everything, from his deepest despair, to moments of relief when the disease has decided to let up, albeit briefly. You will find his story at http://followmylupus.com and he clearly finds writing about what is happening to him has a number of functions. Most importantly, it lightens his own load and gives other lupus sufferers who read it a sense that they are not alone. There is always hope, as Brett says on the site. 'I may be unlucky to have lupus, but I'm lucky to be alive, lucky to have my family and lucky to have my job.'

Lupus in black, Asian and Hispanic populations

One of the many mysteries surrounding lupus is why it is more prevalent in certain ethnic groups. There are numerous theories about this, but few answers. What is known is that black, Asian and Hispanic people have a higher incidence of the condition. In Afro-Caribbean women of child-bearing age the occurrence is as high as one in 250. It is thought that genetics has a big part to play in this – the complex multiple genes that are thought to trigger the disease may be found more often in black and Asian groups.

In the US the incidence of lupus in African American women aged fifteen to sixty-four is one in 245, making it one of the most common chronic diseases in that population. Oddly enough, SLE is currently regarded as a rare disease in Africa, with fewer documented cases there than in the West. There are several possible reasons for this. It could be that the mingling over hundreds of years of African and Caucasian genes has led to a greater genetic susceptibility. Environmental and social factors may have a part to play – poorer communities with limited medical provision are less likely to be able to carry the high cost of diagnosing and treating such a complex and non-specific disease.

A major concern is that awareness of lupus in these ethnic groups is low. Most Afro-Caribbean people will have heard of sickle cell anaemia but not of lupus, despite the fact that SLE is just as much a black person's disease and considerably more common. There is a need for greater education and awareness across the whole population, but these communities should receive special attention. They are the most at risk from lupus, and the condition tends to be more active and aggressive in these groups, commonly attacking major organs like the kidneys and heart.

By the time British-born Diana Reid, whose parents are Jamaican, saw a consultant and got a diagnosis her kidneys had begun to fail. She had been ill for eighteen months without knowing what was wrong. She had been to see doctors at her local GP practice and had been told that the fatigue and swollen joints were to do with stress and she should go home and relax. A simple urine test would have revealed the hidden damage that was going on as lupus attacked her kidneys. Diana, who works as a course coordinator and lives in Beckenham, Kent, in England, says that she was ill for a year and a half before the cause of the problem was pinpointed.

My symptoms started with small rashes all over my body. This was when I was in my early thirties. I would itch like mad, and then my fingers started to tingle. Gradually I developed other problems. I became really tired and my ankles would swell up.

159

Then I started to have an allergic reaction to certain food. My body would react within a couple of minutes – my face, lips, fingers, feet, all of me – would swell. At one point I would become scared if I ate anything with sugar, salt or glucose in it. I was worried that I might suddenly have a bad reaction. It made me look like a monster.

Then I developed double vision and mental confusion. I used to travel to work in the West End of London and just before I got there I would realise that I didn't know where I was heading; I had lost my sense of direction. It really freaked me out but I was too worried about it to tell anyone, especially my work colleagues.

On other occasions the double vision would really play games with me. I would see two of everything and couldn't figure out which was real. Stepping on and off curbs was a nightmare as I didn't know which one of the two I saw was real. If I chose the wrong one I would trip, so I was falling over a lot. It was particularly hard because the doctors did not believe me at first. Then one doctor examined my eyes and saw the changes in my pupils. She got excited, saying this was a rare condition called myasthenia gravis, in which the eye muscles become weak. She told the senior consultant, who also didn't believe it until he saw it for himself.

As well as these problems I found that I had a delayed reaction when trying to pick things up. My movements were slow and I had painful stiff joints. I would get depressed and bad tempered. Now I know that the depression and forgetfulness are symptoms of lupus.

The early days of my illness were hard. I was in a lot of pain in my joints. I was tired and felt so unwell. The symptoms were soul destroying. I thought I was just going mad and a lot of people around me thought that too. So I kept myself to myself. I lost my self-confidence.

When I look back it makes me mad that I had lupus for a year and a half before it was diagnosed. When I showed my doctors the swelling and told them about the tiredness I was told that it was probably due to stress and I should go home and relax. I did this, but I just got worse and worse. In the end I lost faith in them.

A friend finally recommended that I saw a different doctor, who examined me and realised that something was wrong. He took a urine sample and told me that my kidneys were failing, and failing fast. I ended up in hospital and within four weeks they confirmed that I had lupus . . .

The worst times for me were not knowing what was wrong, and then being told that I might have to go on a dialysis machine. I spent two days in Guy's Hospital in London having tests on my kidneys. When I saw the people on the kidney machines I said to myself that there was no way I would end up on one of those things. I started praying and found strength inside to fight this disease.

These days I still experience a little depression and the mood swings. I do get confused and clumsy around the time of my period. At work this is a problem because my brain just slows down and I really get muddled and make a few mistakes. I used to be a high-flyer and quick at spotting errors. Well, things have really changed for me with this illness. I do manage to hide my confusion and memory loss. I can't afford to stop working or go part-time so I just have to get on with it. Looking good despite being ill means people don't treat me differently or guess what is wrong.

Anne-Marie Douglas from Slough, England, aged twenty-six, is another woman who decided to fight back when she became ill with lupus. Anne-Marie, who like Diana has Jamaican parents, realised that few people knew about the disease, and she felt there wasn't enough support for patients. As she is a computer support engineer she had the skills to set up a website for lupus sufferers. The address is www.livingwithlupus.co.uk Anne-Marie also decided to write to newspapers and magazines to tell them her story. *Best* magazine did a feature about her in 2000.

One of the hardest things that Anne-Marie has had to face is the change in her body and her mood swings as a result of steroids. Because she had fluid around the heart and suffers from breathlessness, the amount of exercise she can take is limited.

I used to weigh nine stone, but at one point I went up to twelve stone and that was awful. The steroids also made me grumpy; it is amazing how much you can change as a result of them. I knew this might happen as I had read up as much as I could about the drugs I was taking. When I became short tempered and angry I was a different person and inside I knew my behaviour had changed. Sometimes I find lupus a lonely disease – no one can really understand it unless they have got it. I hate it when people say to me 'It'll be all right', because they don't know how I feel. I decided that setting up a website would be a positive way of coping. It would also allow me to speak to others in the same situation.

When I began talking to other people with lupus as a result of the website, I realised how fortunate I was. There were so many people worse off than me; some who got in touch had lost a loved one to the disease. When I get down about having lupus I remind myself of all those other people and that helps me get through.

As happened for Brett Borowski (*see page 157*), finding a way in which she could talk to many other people who were in the same situation as she was has helped Anne-Marie to come to terms with her condition.

Chapter 11

How Lupus
Affects Families

All chronic diseases can be just as hard on the family as they are on the person with the condition. Whether you are dealing with multiple sclerosis, cancer or rheumatoid arthritis, the disease can tear families apart. Lupus is particularly difficult to cope with as it is unpredictable and fickle. It can range from being virtually unnoticeable to fatal. No one in the family knows how a person with lupus will be from one day to the next, especially when the disease is active. This uncertainty can have a devastating impact. If the person with the disease is the breadwinner it can affect how much money is coming into the house as that person may have to change jobs or leave work completely.

If the person who does most of the chores around the house has lupus they will find it impossible to keep things under control without a great deal of help. Many of the people who suffer from lupus are women in their twenties with young children. This is a particularly harsh reality – the strain on a mother who is not able to deal with her baby or toddler, and on those around her, is immense. Other family members or friends often have to take over the caring role when she is too ill to cope herself.

There is a high chance that a person with lupus will have some neurological involvement, caused either by the disease or by some of the medications prescribed. This can include mood swings, depression, changes in character and odd behaviour, and those involved with the affected person have to be prepared for it.

These pressures can lead to resentment and anger, which in turn can impact on relationships and make life at home hell. Your partner may feel cheated about having married a healthy young woman to find a few years down the line that she has a debilitating incurable disease. Or they might be heroic and give you all the help you need, which makes you feel guilty, angry and cheated of your old healthy life. Your children might find it hard to understand why you are stuck in bed for days on end, and why you don't look the same any more. You may have lost all your hair and put on weight. Their mates can't stay overnight because you can't be exposed to more germs. Your loved ones may have problems believing that you are so sick because lupus is actually making you look glowing and well (this is a characteristic of the disease, *see page 50*).

When it is a child who has lupus, other problems arise – the child coping at school, catching up on missed course work, explaining lupus to their friends, dealing with hospital stays, and not being able to do all the things that other children are doing. It can also be the case that a sick child's siblings suffer as the attention is focused primarily on the sick child. This can lead to long-term resentment and poor sibling relationships.

Support for families

Support networks exist for patients but generally families are overlooked within the medical environment. There is help out there, though, available through charities like Lupus UK and the St Thomas' Lupus Trust (*see* Resources, *page 211*). One of the best ways of dealing with all the family issues that lupus raises is to open up lines of communication – to bring the strong emotions out of the shadows and learn to express them. If family members can let each other know what they are feeling they can put things into perspective and perhaps prevent buried resentment and anger that can gnaw away over years.

Open a dialogue within the household; make the question 'How are you?' count for each member of the family. If any of you feel like being angry, have an outburst and clear the air. If one of you is distressed, share it with your family so they all know how you feel and perhaps why you cry a lot. Communication can make all the difference. Even in the darkest moments, when the pressure is really on, remember that in the vast majority of cases lupus is treatable and the person who has it will get better. What you are going through is therefore temporary. Try and fix your sights on getting through the day and hang on to the knowledge that tomorrow will be different. If the person with lupus is behaving oddly because of the medication they are taking, then a change in dose or drug should alleviate the problem.

Although the system is geared towards patients, as a member of a family of a person who has lupus you shouldn't be afraid to ask for help. At the St Thomas' lupus clinic, for instance, there is a special phone line for patients and their families so they can call for advice. Pressures on time mean you will probably end up leaving a message, but the machines are closely monitored. If you develop a good relationship with the local team you will find that they will also give families this kind of back-up. If not then try the local lupus charity groups. Don't be afraid to reach out for help. There is no shame in being overwhelmed by the destructive nature of lupus and you will find plenty of others in the same boat.

Also learn as much as possible about the condition through books or the Internet, or by becoming involved in the lupus charities. Chatting to others in the same situation can not only make you feel less isolated but also give you important tips on dealing with lupus. If there are deep-seated relationship problems the person with lupus should let their specialist know. They will be able to give advice or steer you in the direction of a clinical psychologist or psychiatrist who is familiar with lupus and can provide coping strategies to get you through the bad times.

Family members can be brought along to clinics – although not en masse! This can help them get a grasp of what the disease is about. They can hear what the doctors have to say and see that there is a lot that can be done for the patient. They can talk to team members and get guidance on how to give the best support. This is also a good opportunity for family members to develop a close relationship with the medical team.

The crucial message for families and friends of lupus sufferers is 'You are not alone'. Although the system doesn't focus on how the disease has affected you there is help out there; you just have to look for it. See Resources (*page 211*) for names and addresses of organisations and websites that you are likely to find useful.

Sex and lupus

This is a subject that is rarely dealt with in any formal way in clinics or during medical appointments, despite the fact that lupus can have a major effect on a couple's sex life. It's a concern that there is little research available on this issue to date, even though a couple whose sex life has died a death are likely to have real problems with their relationship. Burying this issue will not make it go away. The chances are that it will crop up time and time again until you do something about it.

Do not be afraid to talk to your specialist if you are having sexual problems. When you are treated you should be dealt with as a whole person, not just as someone with lupus. Your general welfare should be taken into account and a breakdown in your relationship will have a profound impact on your well-being.

There are particular problems that can occur with lupus and the related diseases. For instance, Sjogren's syndrome (*see page 58*) can cause vaginal dryness, so intercourse may be uncomfortable without some kind of lubrication. There are plenty of lubricants available over the counter at chemists or on prescription. Lupus can cause vaginal ulcers, which are unpleasant and can be painful during sex. They should respond to the treatment you are on for other lupus symptoms. If they do not, let your doctor know.

When you have sore joints probably the last thing you feel like doing is engaging in some bedroom gymnastics, but this doesn't mean that you should avoid having sex altogether. It doesn't have to be a marathon; it can be gentle and paced to suit how you feel. The key once again is communication. Few couples discuss their sex lives with each other, never mind complete strangers, but with a chronic illness you have to overcome the fear of dealing with this issue. In fact, having a good sex life will help make you feel better all around. It will boost your mood and improve your self-esteem – two vital antidotes to having a chronic disease.

There are sex counsellors whom you can see, although you might have to pay for the service. As with so many things in lupus the best course of action is to broach the subject with your medical team. If you feel embarrassed about raising it with your consultant, have a word with the clinic nurse, who will be familiar with these problems and will be able to give you some guidance on how best to get help.

Lupus and bereavement

This is the darkest side of lupus, which no one is keen to discuss. Doctors are reluctant to put too much emphasis on the potentially fatal nature of lupus as the number of patients who die from the disease is relatively few. Quite under-standably, they do not want to frighten people who have this condition as the vast majority will live a relatively normal life once they get a diagnosis and treatment. The fact remains, however, that despite the considerable advances in treat-ment, SLE can be fatal. It is therefore important to know and understand this aspect of the condition and the impact it has on families and friends.

Two age groups have the highest mortality rates: the teens and early twenties, and people over fifty. In the younger age group most deaths are among females. Lupus can be particularly brutal in this age group and target major organs and the central nervous system. In the over fifties deaths are usually due to a number of factors. They may be a result of organs being permanently damaged due to the effects of the lupus over many years, or to the cumulative impact of the side effects caused by long-term medication. For instance, steroids taken over many years, especially when they have been used in high doses, can affect the heart and fur up the arteries, leading to cardiac problems.

Any age group, however, can be affected. While researching this book I came across a family whose eleven-year-old daughter had died as a result of a catastrophic lupus flare. She developed difficulty breathing, some major organs 'shut down' and she went into a coma from which she did not recover. The girl was receiving treatment for lupus symptoms, but sometimes the disease can be so aggressive and out of control that there is little doctors can do.

Carrie from Birmingham had been ill since she was fourteen, but she didn't get a diagnosis for her array of symptoms until she was seventeen. Sadly, within days of finding out she had lupus, Carrie had a number of seizures. The lupus had attacked her brain, lungs and heart. Despite attempts to revive her, Carrie did not pull through. Her family felt that if she had got a diagnosis sooner she might still be with them. It's impossible to know whether or not that is the case, but we do know that the majority of patients have a hard time getting a diagnosis because of the lack of awareness about lupus. Losing a loved one is devastating; losing someone to a disease where treatment might have been successful if there had been greater awareness and an earlier diagnosis must be almost unbearable.

It is hard to get firm figures on the numbers of deaths in the United Kingdom. As with so many things to do with lupus there is limited information available. The lupus clinic at St Thomas' Hospital has 2,500 patients on its register and roughly five people die each year, but obviously that does not give an accurate figure for the wider population. It only gives an idea of the numbers of deaths within a group of people who have been so unwell with lupus that they have been referred to a specialist clinic. Among people with a diagnosis the mortality rate is low – they know what they have and the more sophisticated specialist treatments are literally lifesavers.

It is, however, hard to gauge what impact undetected lupus has on mortality across the population. SLE is rarely written on a death certificate, and a cause of death might be written down as, say, kidney failure – with no indication that this was due to lupus. The doctor writing the certificate might not even know that this disease was present.

The United States is some way ahead of the United Kingdom in terms of keeping statistics for lupus. A report by the American Centers for Disease Control and Prevention published in July 2002 showed that the death rate from SLE was rising. It looked at a period from 1979 to 1998. The study found that the annual number of deaths from lupus climbed from 879 in 1979 to 1,406 in 1998. More than a third of these deaths occurred in people aged between fifteen and forty-four.

The increase sounds alarming and American lupus charities used them to get headlines and thereby raise awareness of the disease. However, the report had a number of limitations. Firstly, looking at death certificates to get lupus figures is misleading. The figures are likely to be much higher because as mentioned above, SLE can contribute to a death but not be mentioned on the certificate. The data may also be affected by the over or under diagnosis because of the difficulties in spotting lupus.

Dr Bob Lahita of Jersey City Hospital in the US estimates that among his patients five in a hundred die from SLE each year, but once again the people he sees are those with diagnosed lupus, so this does not give a true picture for the wider population.

The number of deaths from lupus has dropped dramatically since I first became involved in this field in 1975. This is due to better diagnosis and the way we use drugs these days. The highest mortality rate is among young women. The older woman who dies is not that common. Years ago the problems were related to immuno-suppression. Today patients live on for a long time and the biggest concern is athrosclerotic cardiovascular disease. That is a major concern in this population.

Death certificates are very interesting in relation to lupus. I sign a lot of death certificates and I never really know what the patient's complications were. So we say cardiopulmonary failure but it can be cardiopulmonary failure because of SLE. It can be renal fail-ure which led to cardiopulmonary failure. Looking at death certifi-cates is not a way to get a true figure of who dies from lupus. We obviously have our own figures here as we monitor our patients, and looking at that I would say that we lose about fifty people per thousand.

Janet Dean, the Labour MP for Burton, Lancashire, in England, has suffered more than most due to lupus. First her mother died of the disease after years of illness. Thirteen years later her husband Alan, whom she describes as her soulmate, died suddenly of a heart attack after having lupus for eighteen years. Janet and her two daughters Carol and Sandra have had a lifetime of learning how to cope with SLE. In the face of tremendous loss the three have adopted the attitude 'We know we just have to get on with life'.

Janet says:

When mum was eventually diagnosed I had to have the condition written down to know even how you said it. I had never heard of it before. I couldn't remember a time when mum wasn't ill. She developed symptoms just after I was born, when she was thirty-eight. Mum had so many things wrong with her – arthritis, pleurisy, Raynaud's and headaches. We didn't get a diagnosis, though, for twenty-one years, when mum was fifty-nine. By that time the lupus had affected her heart; she was a semi-invalid and she then developed diabetes as a result of the steroid treatments she had been having. However, I think she was relieved to have a name for what was wrong. We tried to find out what we could about the disease, which was difficult as there wasn't much information available in 1970. With lupus there is a sense of isolation, which is why groups like Lupus UK are so important.

For Janet and her young family worse was yet to come. In 1976 her husband Alan, a railway clerk and local councillor, became unwell.

Alan was exhausted. We went to the doctor, who was a locum, and he said you either have flu or a very serious disease. Given the choice you would go for the flu but as it turned out that was one of the initial symptoms of lupus. At that stage we had no idea that he was suffering from the same condition as Mum.

Over the next two years Alan got worse. He developed fevers and fatigue, and was diagnosed with gout and depression. Then in the autumn of 1978 things got dramatically worse. He became more and more ill with painful joints, mouth ulcers and skin lesions. There was also some brain involvement; he was confused and not like himself. Alan was hallucinating, speaking to people who weren't there. At the

173

time we thought it was to do with his fever, but with hind-sight you can see it was part of lupus.

I can remember thinking at one point that Alan looked just like my mother, or the symptoms were just like my mother's. Even when I thought that, though, I couldn't really believe that he could have the same condition.

They admitted Alan to hospital and he was desperately ill. He had a grand mal seizure, and was in hospital for thirteen weeks in total. Alan had other symptoms, like short-term memory problems, tics and twitches, and loss of sight, for short periods of time.

There are things you don't say but at the time I feared he might die. In the three months he was in the Derbyshire Royal Infirmary I took the girls with me to see him a lot of the time. They were six and eight at the time. We were fortu-nate because Alan worked on the railway so we had free travel. It was winter and there I was with these two little tots travelling back and forth to hospital – we only missed a few days out of a hundred. All the time there was the anxiety that the treatment wasn't going to work.

The consultant said Alan had 'sticky blood' [Hughes syndrome], but in 1978 they didn't know the relevance of that. Today he would be on anticoagulants and he wouldn't need the same high dose of steroids. Alan's symptoms were much more dramatic than my mother's with the cerebral involvement and the terrible pains and stiffness. From being six foot and broad he went to twelve stone; he looked terribly ill at that point, although later, with treatment, he looked well – as many people with lupus do.

Alan always thought he was a success story, right up to his death, because the initial dramatic condition had been treated and he had recovered and gone on to do so much. He went back to work, initially part-time, then full-time, but not on shifts any more. He stood for re-election to the council, and for a by-election in 1980. He was never 100 per cent well, though – he had his good days and his bad days. He got tired and felt sheer exhaustion and joint pains. He had one thing or another. He always felt that the cerebral involvement had left him not quite as sharp as he had been, but he was obviously still able to cope. He went on to become mayor and then chair of East Staffordshire District Council.

My two girls have just grown up with lupus. Carol was a babe in arms when my mother was diagnosed. Lupus became part of family life. It did restrict us as a family – for instance, we would go for holidays in Britain and not abroad because Alan was photosensitive. Early on the girls couldn't understand why I would insist that their friends kept away if they had colds or infections. They thought I was being quite hard as a parent, but now they understand why I didn't want Alan to be exposed to those germs.

Alan died suddenly in 1994 – he was only forty-six. He had been having some pain and was tired, and we thought it was a flare of lupus. We didn't know he had a heart condition.

Alan loved to be out and about, and on this particular day he went off to see the football team Crewe Alexandra play at Rotherham. He was on his way home, at Meadowhall Railway Station, when he collapsed and died on the platform. It's hard to describe the trauma of the police knocking on the door with such terrible news. It was so unexpected. By the time my daughters and I went up to Sheffield on the Monday to iden-tify the body the post mortem had been done. There was therefore no opportunity to establish whether the heart attack was caused by the condition or by years of treatment.

My mother's death was a sad loss, but when she died in 1981, living to the age of seventy was considered a good long life. To lose Alan, on the other hand, when he was just forty-six and had been my soulmate for most of my life, was devastating. I only got through by keeping busy. I decided I would stand for Parliament if the party wanted me and it did. I had stood for selection in the 1992 election, and when Alan died I decided to put my name forward again. My great interest in politics and the support of my family and friends pulled me through.

When Alan was alive we did some work towards raising awareness locally, and although we joined Lupus UK nationally we didn't get involved at a regional level. Now I have set up the All Party Parliamentary Group for Lupus in Parliament to put lupus on the map and help raise the profile of lupus with the Department of Health.

You always think 'Could I have done more or said more?' But you can't allow yourself to dwell on that. At least Mum and Alan had a diagnosis. Without that and the dedication of the medical profession, neither of them would have survived so long.

Lupus is a condition that can either drive you apart or bring you closer. In our case it brought Alan and me closer – we loved to spend time with each other. We were at school together and grew up together, and at least I have my memories.

Chapter 12

Towards a Diagnosis: An Action Plan

Hundreds of kind and courageous people volunteered to be part of this book in person, or by post, email or phone. They were prompted to volunteer because they felt there was a desperate need to increase awareness of lupus. I would estimate that at least 95 per cent of them had a terrible struggle to get a diagnosis. Some had been through a lifetime of pain and suffering, made worse by disbelief and ignorance, while others were still awaiting the diagnosis that would free them from the distress of not knowing.

There are plenty of reasons why these problems arise, most of which have been dealt with earlier. They boil down to ignorance of the condition and the complex and non-specific nature of SLE. Spotting it is difficult and can be a long process. The key is for lupus to be considered as a possible diagnosis in the first place. For that to happen your doctor has to have a certain degree of awareness and a grasp of the symptoms. Many people with lupus have told me how they had to 'train their doctor' about lupus.

It would be wrong and unhelpful to come down too hard on doctors. They have an uphill struggle to pin down this condition and in general practice they do not have the tools, time or expertise to deliver a conclusive diagnosis of lupus. Then again there are plenty of patients who feel that their primary care was flawed and that obvious signs were missed in the early stages. Staying bitter against the medical profession won't get you very far – you need the doctors. If you feel there really was some negligence, talk to a solicitor. If you don't, you should move on and save your energy for fighting the real enemy – lupus. Concentrate on getting the lupus under control and getting on with your life.

Seeing a doctor

No one likes having to see a doctor. Sitting in a packed clinic feeling that your fate is in someone else's hands is disconcerting and frightening. In lupus this is made harder by the fact that you are likely to have been unwell for some time with all sorts of odd symptoms that appear to be unconnected. You might have had repeated appointments without getting a diagnosis, and in some cases this could have gone on for years. You could be feeling disheartened because all the tests have come back negative. The list of things wrong might be so long that even you begin to doubt yourself. So you start at a disadvantage, because you are uncertain and scared. You have already planted the seed in your own mind that you might be a hypochondriac, accompanied by the concern that you will walk out of the appointment you have waited for months to get still feeling dreadful and none the wiser.

At the other end of the spectrum you might just be starting out on your lupus journey, so you are not used to seeing doctors. The environment is alien, the language incomprehensible. More worrying still is if you are seeing a specialist – an 'ologist' – for the first time; they can seem even more aloof and dismissive.

There are a number of things you can do to make the whole thing less of an ordeal and to make the appointment count. You have to remember that however high powered doctors may be, they are flesh and blood like the rest of us. Don't let the white coat and stethoscope fool you. A trick I use to make doctors less scary is to conjure up a scene from the 1954 classic comedy film *Doctor in the House*. It's the bit where the pompous chief surgeon – Sir Lancelot Spratt, played by James Robertson Justice – bullies his group of medical students on a ward round. He gathers them around a hospital bed and barks at them to tell him what is wrong with the patient. Of course, the young medics don't have a clue and are generally more interested in the nurses than the patients. The men in white coats – and it was all men as I recall – struggle unsuccessfully to come up with a diagnosis. Their saviour is the middle-aged patient they are examining. He comes to the rescue by giving them broad hints as to what is wrong with him and pointing to the relevant parts of his anatomy.

The scene is a reminder that it is often the patient who knows their condition better than the doctors. They are the ones who hold the vital clues as to what is wrong, and the first thing a good doctor will do is listen to the patient and take a comprehensive medical and social history. Even though doctors appear to have your life in their hands, in the end the outcome is up to you – after all it is your body. Never be afraid of your doctor, whether it is your own GP or a consultant. If you do feel unhappy with the way you are being treated you can ask to see a different person. I know that when you are very sick you don't feel much like fighting the system, but you might just have to dig deep and find that extra bit of strength. Perhaps someone close to you could help.

There are various things you can do to make the process less bewildering and stressful. A bit of focused preparation will assist in getting what you need from the experts.

Make every moment of your appointment count

In the lupus world there are painfully few medical specialists who are up to speed with the latest tests and treatments. The knock-on effect for the patient is that you will have had to wait a long time, probably months, to see the right people. When you do eventually get in front of them they will be under a tremendous amount of pressure as they work their way through heavily booked clinics. So you must try to make every moment count.

Don't go alone

Try to bring someone with you. It could be your partner, a family member or a friend. A second pair of eyes and ears will help to ensure that you remember what the doctor said – sometimes you can get into such a state that you miss great chunks of their wise words. It can happen to us all. Fear can make you temporarily deaf and dumb, so having someone there who isn't in the firing line and won't suffer a bout of amnesia really does help.

It is also good to have moral support on hand. You can never be 100 per cent sure about the outcome of an appointment. You might trot off home with a prescription or be sent for blood tests, or the doctor may decide that they want to admit you to hospital straight from the clinic.

Keep a diary

It is important to keep a diary of your illness. A doctor's first question is often, 'When did you first feel unwell?' This is likely to be followed by, 'Can you describe how you felt and what the symptoms were?' and 'How have you been since then?' Doctors need to work like detectives. They have to piece together the evidence and the timescale of an illness to catch the culprit. As in a police investigation, timing can be crucial to the case, especially where there are so many different clues and incidents. If you can have answers at the ready it will speed things up.

List your symptoms

Writing down a list of current symptoms is important in lupus. This is because so many people with lupus have had a considerable number of things wrong with them. The doctor will want to know what the most recent symptoms are. I used to find that sitting there and going through a great long list was embarrassing, so I would type out my 'summary of symptoms' to hand to the consultant. That way I didn't forget anything and didn't have to drone on. The young student doctors who invariably sat in on these sessions would go wide-eyed and look terribly impressed by the number and variety of things that were wrong with me – that's something that is only amusing in retrospect.

Maintain a visual record

During a session with the doctor you are likely to have a physical examination. With lupus this is essential – 'clinical observations' can reveal so much. Lupus can manifest itself in so many ways that you are unlikely to be aware of all the telltale signs, but the lupus specialists will be. A trained eye will spot changes in skin colour and condition, for instance, or rashes and distorted joints that have crept up on you so slowly that you weren't even aware of them. With lupus the results of a physical examination are crucial and can be as important as blood tests, although both are usually used to make a diagnosis and decide on treatment. Sometimes the wait to see a specialist is so long that rashes and lesions can come and go. If, therefore, you can get your hands on a camera, photograph the affected area and bring the evidence along to your appointment.

Take notes on your medication

Maintain a record of any medication you are prescribed. If you know what drugs and doses you are on this will save you time when you are talking to the doctor in future. If you have those details written down it will help if your mind goes blank. Having this information will also enable you to read up on the medication in medical reference books or on the Internet in your own time.

Take notes during your appointment

It is important to always take notes during a session with the specialist. If you have someone with you, ask them to jot down what they can. Alternatively you could record the most important part of the session if the consultant doesn't mind you doing this. It is very common for a patient to get flustered, especially if lots of medical terms are being used. A doctor will usually try and explain what is being said, but in the panic of the moment it is possible for difficult medical names to be wiped immediately from your memory. For instance, if your consultant says that you have 'antiphospholipid antibodies', the chances are that within seconds of leaving the consulting room you will have no idea what they said. This won't be because you aren't clever, but because you are not a doctor and have other things on your mind.

If you have a record of what is said you can look things up later in medical publications or on the Internet. No matter how well read you are about lupus, the range of symptoms and treatments is such that you cannot always know what the doctor is talking about during a consultation.

Record your medical history

Give your medical history some thought before the appointment, and make sure you have dates and symptoms jotted down. For instance, the doctor will want to know about any pregnancies or miscarriages, any previous autoimmune problems, or whether you had any growing pains or glandular fever when you were younger. Was there anything odd about your health when you were growing up? Have you had a history of headaches or migraine, blood clots or high blood pressure? If you can spend some time thinking about your past medical history before you see the doctor this will help. It is difficult to bring these things to mind on the spur of the moment when you feel stressed and under pressure.

Find out your family's medical history

Because lupus has a genetic component, the doctor will want to explore your family's medical history. You are likely to be asked whether there is a history in your family of thrombosis, immune conditions like arthritis or ME, joint problems, stroke, heart attack, chronic fatigue or miscarriage. Obviously, you can't canvass your family members once you are at the clinic, so spend a bit of time asking them about any known illnesses across the most recent generations before you come for the appointment.

Bring a list of questions

You are highly likely to have many of your own questions. Write them down before you see the doctor. Put them in order of importance in case you don't have time to ask them all. Remember to write down the answers, if not in full then just the key points, and get the spellings for any medical words that you don't understand so that you can look them up later. If you have read up about lupus you will be familiar with some of the terms used in relation to the disease. If you don't understand a description, ask the doctor to explain further; they are there to help you.

Know your subject

Knowing as much as you can about this condition will help you to control it and live as normal a life as the rest of the population. In my experience doctors in this field respond well to patients who have learned as much as they can about lupus. It makes their job easier if you have a grasp of what they are looking for and what treatments they will use. Information on further contacts and other publications is given in Resources (*see page 211*).

To summarise . . .

- Ensure that you make your visit count.

- Bring a relative or friend.

- Keep a diary of your illness and use it at your appointment.

- List your symptoms both past and present. Try to recall the sequence of events: when different symptoms appeared, for how long and how did they affect you? Describe the symptoms to the doctor.

- Take a photograph of any rashes or lesions and show this to the doctor.

- Keep your own record of your medication – find out the details at your appointment.

- During your appointment, take notes or record what the doctor says.

- Write out your own medical history, and have this to hand at your appointment.

- Get a family medical history together and pass any relevant information to the doctor.

- Write down questions to ask the doctor.

- Find out as much as you can about lupus before your appointment.

Chapter 13

You Are Not Alone

In this chapter you will see that if you have lupus you are in good company. Although most people are only just beginning to recognise the existence of lupus, the condition has actually been around for thousands of years. Very early medical descriptions of a disease that caused severe skin damage, fever and joint pain go back to ancient Greece. Hippocrates, the Greek physician born in 460 BC, wrote about people who had severe red ulcerating lesions to the skin. Lupus is Latin for 'wolf'; its usage in relation to a medical condition first appeared in the thirteenth century in work by a physician called Rogerius. Later on, in the early 1500s, it was used by Paracelsus. They both mentioned 'lupus' to describe facial skin damage.

No one is sure why this condition came to be named after a wolf, although there are two popular theories. One theory is that it referred to the rash that appeared to eat away at the skin, leaving terrible scarring resembling injuries that could be sustained as a result of being attacked by a wolf. The other explanation is that the frightening appearance of some people with lupus made them resemble a wolf, in particular the malar rash across the cheeks and nose. In some communities there were even superstitions about a link with werewolves.

Lupus in medicine

The name lupus was originally used for a broad spectrum of conditions. There was no specific illness, and the symptoms the term embraced were mainly to do with the skin. It was only relatively recently – in 1851 – that the definition became more precise. This was when the French doctor Pierre Cazanave identified three different types of lupus, and he was the first to use the term 'lupus erythematosus'. The next major step came from the renowned Canadian physician Sir William Osler at the turn of the last century. He wrote a series of papers on lupus erythematosus that demonstrated internal organs could be involved, including the heart, kidneys and central nervous system. He highlighted the fact that lupus could be 'systemic' – that it could affect the whole body rather than just one part of it. Dr Osler also wrote that a special feature of the disease was that it could relapse, with flares recurring over a period of months or years. This work set the foundation for advances in the identification of lupus, both SLE and discoid. In the 1930s and 1940s doctors began to identify common aspects of the disease in patients, and this was a step towards putting together criteria for lupus.

The first useful test for lupus came in the 1920s, when doctors recognised that a 'false positive' blood test for syphilis would often point to the presence of SLE, although this was not specific for lupus and had to be used in conjunction with other tests. Perhaps the most important breakthrough came in 1948 with the development of the first blood test actually for lupus. Pathologists at the Mayo Clinic in the US spotted an oddly shaped white blood cell in the bone marrow samples of lupus patients. They published their findings and called the cell the 'LE', or 'lupus erythematosus', cell. The test wasn't conclusive, but it was a great deal more precise than the syphilis test. At about the same time Dr Phillip Hench made his Nobel-prize-winning discovery that steroids could be used to treat joint inflammation (*see page 84*).

Since the groundbreaking work by the Mayo Clinic, blood tests have been refined and broadened. In the 1950s and 1960s, work focused on antibodies. So called 'fluorescent tests' were developed to detect antibodies that attacked the nucleus of cells – the ANA. It was found that the blood of lupus patients could often be characterised by certain anti-bodies being present – in particular those that work against the 'double-helix' DNA. This led to a test that measured the anti-DNA antibodies. It proved to be an excellent tool for diagnosing SLE and is used routinely today (*see page 66*).

Lupus and some historical figures

It is possible to see the footprint of lupus throughout history, in particular by looking at high-profile figures whose lives, health and deaths have been closely charted by histo-rians. Because lupus was not identified as a multi-organ disease until relatively recently it does not appear in medical records by name, but the symptoms speak for themselves. You have to weigh up the evidence, a bit like a detective. Although it is impossible to be certain whether some famous historical figures had lupus, Queen Anne's case was relatively clear cut.

Queen Anne, British monarch

One of the most prominent historical figures suspected of having lupus is Queen Anne, the last of the Stuart monarchs.

There is strong evidence that she died as a result of SLE and that she also had Hughes syndrome.

Queen Anne was born in 1665, the younger daughter of King James II. Records show that Anne was a sickly child, and in later life she was said to suffer from porphyria. This is a rare genetic blood disorder that can lead to skin rashes and blistering when the affected person is exposed to sunlight, and to abdominal pain and disturbances of the nervous system. On examining the evidence, however, this diagnosis does not stand, as it fails to explain the variety and complexity of the Queen's ailments. In particular, porphyria does not affect pregnancy, and poor Queen Anne had terrible problems in this department.

Anne married Prince George of Denmark when she was just eighteen and proceeded to do her duty by attempting to produce an heir to the throne, thereby securing the Stuart line. She became pregnant the year after her marriage and there was great hope in royal circles that this meant she was highly fertile. The first inkling that things would not go to plan came with the stillbirth of Anne's baby girl in May 1684.

Over a period of eighteen years Anne is known to have had at least seventeen pregnancies. Of these there were five live births, one stillbirth and eleven miscarriages. The only child to live for any length of time was Duke William of Gloucester. He was unwell for much of his life; his head was enlarged with arrested hydrocephalus – which means he had increased fluid around the brain. He died a few days after his eleventh birthday from pneumonia, which was common in those days.

It is hard to get a full picture of all of Anne's pregnancies, but there is enough detail around to show that the majority of the miscarriages came in later pregnancy. They were certainly far enough down the line for the sex of the foetus to be clear, so she would probably have been well into the second trimester. Here are the dates and other information that have survived in the historical record.

Date		Offspring
1684	12 May	Stillborn daughter
1685	2 June–8 February 1687	Mary or Marie
1686	2 June–2 February 1687	Anne Sophia
1687	20 January–4 February	Miscarriage
1688	October	Miscarriage, male
1689	24 July–30 July 1700	William Duke of Gloucester
1690	14 October– died after two hours	Mary (two months premature)
1692	17 April– died after a few minutes	George
1693	23 March	Miscarriage, female
1694	21 January	Miscarriage
1696	18 February	Miscarriage, female
1696	20 September	Double miscarriage
1697	25 March	Miscarriage
1697	December	Miscarriage
1698	15 September	Miscarriage, male
1700	25 January	Miscarriage, male

This must have been devastating for Queen Anne, especially as she had to contend with her own poor health while trying desperately to have children. She has often been criticised by historians for not being a more powerful monarch, but it is hardly surprising that she might have seemed a bit preoccupied when you consider the obstetric nightmare she struggled through and the pressure she was under to give the nation a future monarch.

Queen Anne had a lifetime of ill health. She was often unable to move and was bedridden. She had uncomfortable rashes, severe arthritic pain and swollen joints. Portraits of Anne show the high red, almost puce colour of her face. Despite her illness, though, she had a good appetite, which further damaged her health in later years as she became obese and rarely took any exercise.

These days a specialist would immediately test for SLE, and the obstetric history would certainly lead to tests for antiphospholipid antibodies. After years of speculation about Queen Anne's health there is a growing body of thought that supports the view that she had SLE and Hughes syndrome. A recent book (*The Sickly Stuarts*) by Frederick Holmes, emeritus professor of medicine at the University of Kansas Medical Center in the US, carefully examines the evidence, including the post mortem on the Queen and reports from the time. He shares the view that lupus was the culprit:

Systemic lupus erythematosus remains the best explanation for Anne's ill-starred obstetric history and the disabling rheumatic disease she suffered in the last decade or so of her life. This is in agreement with the opinions expressed by Emson (H.E. Emson, Canadian pathologist who assessed Anne's obstetric problems in 1992) and also serves the principle of adducing one disease to explain all of Anne's medical problems . . . it is certain that Anne had systemic lupus erythematosus and that the progression of this disease led to her premature death from a cerebrovascular event – a stroke – common among sufferers of this disease.

Professor Holmes also states:

Pregnancy in disseminated lupus erythematosus, particularly in the presence of the antiphospholipid antibody, is associated with

191

miscarriage, placental damage and insufficiency and foetal death. In modern times this antibody can be identified easily in some women who have lost more than one pregnancy, and among the treatment options to sustain subsequent pregnancies is a single aspirin tablet taken daily. In all likelihood in the early eighteenth century the equivalent was actually available as salicylic acid in herbal preparations containing willow bark, although its efficacy in Anne's condition could not have been known at the time . . . clearly Anne had the antiphospholipid antibody.

The Queen died in 1714; the days leading up to her death saw her racked with pain, slipping in and out of consciousness. When she was lucid she complained of a severe headache and nausea and suffered vomiting. It appears that there was damage to the brain due to a stroke that could have resulted from clotting brought on by Hughes syndrome, although years of untreated lupus is also likely to have played a part in causing vascular damage and leading to her death.

What is particularly interesting is that Anne's elder sister Mary also had obstetric problems, having two miscarriages and then no further pregnancies. The sisters' mother, Anne, had eight pregnancies. Obviously the two girls survived to adulthood, but of the others only two sons lived for any length of time, both dying at the age of four. We know there is a genetic link in lupus, so it isn't beyond possibility that SLE was responsible for health problems seen in a number of generations of Stuarts.

If Anne had lived today she would have had a full screen for lupus and Hughes syndrome. If these conditions were confirmed and she received the correct treatment her chances of having an heir would have been as high as 80 per cent, and the quality of her life and health would have improved dramatically. The Stuart line would have been secured and the British monarchy may have taken quite a different course.

Ludwig van Beethoven, composer

Ludwig van Beethoven's case is less clear than that of Queen Anne. Arguments have raged from even before his death as to what was behind the poor state of his health. What caused his deafness, heightened facial colouring, gut problems, joint pain, odd behavioural changes and so on? Beethoven himself was tortured by the uncertainty of what ailed him. He asked that after his death a professor whom he knew should carry out a post mortem to resolve the question. Hundreds of years later that question remains unanswered.

One strange aspect of lupus is that it does not affect the liver, so the fact that doctors at the time of Beethoven's death recorded that he died of liver failure due to cirrhosis might appear to rule out SLE. It is, however, known that Beethoven was a heavy drinker for thirty years or so and that could have contributed to the liver problems. He certainly had a broad spectrum of health problems – for instance deafness, which could have been due to a thickening of the bone in his middle ear; this was again not lupus. There were, however, other symptoms which some doctors think point to autoimmune problems.

Beethoven had facial scarring, said to be from a childhood illness, but these markings could have been a rash linked with SLE. He had arthritis that physicians said was rheumatism, and he was reported to have had repeated bouts of rheumatic fever. High temperatures, and swollen hands and joints, are all symptoms seen in lupus. Another aspect of Beethoven's condition – his behavioural problems – is something that hasn't been fully considered before in the context of his illness. Perhaps it should be now, especially as we know that 90 per cent of lupus sufferers have some kind of neurological involvement, from mild depression to psychosis. This might explain some of Beethoven's more excessive mood swings.

Consultant physician Edward Larkin supported the view that the composer had autoimmune problems when he wrote in the medical section in the book *Beethoven – the Last Decade*, in 1970:

Beethoven may well have had a specific form of immunopathic disease known as systemic lupus erythematosus, which typically commences in early adult life with a fever accompanied by mental confusion. Typical symptoms are destructive rash and redness of the butterfly area of the face. Any of the immunopathic disorders may occur, notably colitis. The excellent life mask of 1812 shows an elongated atrophic scar particularly suggestive of lupus. The portraits clearly show flushing of the cheekbones and nose.

Hugh Gaitskell, politician

Lupus had a hand in changing the course of history for the British Labour party. The formidable Labour leader in the 1950s, Hugh Todd Gaitskell, died unexpectedly in 1963 at the age of fifty-seven. This was a particularly cruel death for a career politician who was at the peak of his powers and had Number Ten directly in his sights. As it was, Gaitskell's death cleared the way for the young Harold Wilson to lead the party to electoral victory.

Hugh Gaitskell's death was a mystery – there was even some suggestion that he had been assassinated by the KGB with ricin poison. He died within weeks and little information was made available at the time as to why. The truth is that he died as a result of an aggressive flare of SLE that led to kidney failure. His family kept this a secret at the time, perhaps because no one knew about lupus in the 1960s. His widow Dora did confirm that he had lupus when she was approached many years ago by a member of Lupus UK.

Mary Flannery O'Connor, US writer

Mary Flannery O'Connor, a woman regarded as one of the most important voices in American literature, lost her battle against lupus at the age of thirty-nine. The author of *A Good Man Is Hard to Find* fought for years against SLE, endeavouring to write as much as she could when she was in good health. She knew, however, what fate had in store as her father had died of lupus when she was twenty-nine years old.

Jack London, US writer

More controversial is the view that Jack London, the novelist and short-story writer who was wowing the US from California in the 1900s, died as a result of lupus symptoms. He was just forty years old and initially his death in 1916 was put down to suicide due to a morphine overdose. This theory has been challenged recently in light of evidence that he had suffered for years with an excruciatingly painful kidney condition that could have been lupus. The morphine was to relieve the pain. If he did have SLE how ironic it is that a number of his major works included wolves and that the dream home he built in California was called Wolf House.

The rich and famous get it too

Lupus recognises no social barriers. It can strike at any part of the community. However, there are differences in how various communities are equipped to detect and cope with the disease. Among the wealthy diagnosis and expensive drugs are not an issue, but that doesn't bring with it immunity. Nor does celebrity.

One of the most effective campaigners for awareness about lupus in the United States is Howie Dorough, a member of the band Backstreet Boys. His sister Caroline died from lupus in 1998. Since then Howie has dedicated much of his time to fighting the disease. He has set up a foundation and raised millions of dollars to help promote awareness, to support patients who cannot afford treatment and to fund research.

Other names in the 'lupus hall of fame' include the British pop star Seal, who is reported to have discoid lupus that has marked his skin, and the opera singer Jessie Norman has lupus and dedicates time to raising awareness of the condition. The former singer from the band Eternal, Kelle Bryan, has talked about how she copes with having lupus, although she has regretted being so open. After she spoke out on a television show the headlines in the national newspapers wrongly implied that she was going to die and had been told she would never sing again. She was distressed by the exaggerated reporting and hasn't spoken publicly about lupus since.

Michael Wayne, the eldest son of the film star John Wayne, died in the spring of 2003 of heart failure as a result of complications from lupus. Michael Wayne, who produced some of his famous father's Westerns, was sixty-eight years old and had struggled with the disease for some time.

Michael Jackson, US singer

Michael Jackson is believed to have discoid lupus. Dr Bob Lahita treated the star in hospital in New Jersey after Jackson was burned while filming an advert. Dr Lahita says the lesions from lupus were found on his scalp, where the hair had burned away.

Michael Jackson has discoid lupus and vitiligo, which is also autoimmune. He definitely has it – I actually saw it. Another doctor and myself discovered the discoid lupus after Michael's hair caught on fire during a Coca-Cola commercial. The accident had damaged his hair and exposed his scalp. This is where we saw the lesions. I don't believe he knew he had discoid lupus up to that time; all he knew was that he had vitiligo. He is very light sensitive.

Currently Michael Jackson has said publicly only that he has vitiligo, although members of his family confirm that he also has skin lupus.

Elaine Paige, British singer

It is hard for anyone to cope with an illness like lupus, but it can be especially difficult for performers who rely on physical fitness to do their jobs. Life can be tough on a dancer who has demanding routines to do each night, but at the same time is dealing with joint swelling and pain. The show must go on, but it comes at a cost.

Elaine Paige, one of Britain's foremost female performers, knows first-hand how hard this can be. Elaine, who is known for her major roles in hit musicals like *Evita, Cats, Piaf, Sunset Boulevard* and *The King and I*, suffers from a mild form of lupus. Although she has supported lupus charities for a number of years she has always steered clear of talking publicly about how the condition affected her – that is until now.

Elaine is one of the 'lucky ones' when it comes to lupus, as her condition is now well under control and does not affect her work on stage. There was a time back in 1989 when her life was suddenly plunged into uncertainty. Elaine went through what so many people with lupus do – the distress of not knowing what was wrong.

Lupus affected me in the most devastating way. I was rehearsing for Anything Goes *at the Prince Edward Theatre in 1989. It was a tough schedule and a very physical show and I was co-producing so there was quite a lot of stress. In the middle of rehearsals I caught a cold though it developed into what seemed like flu symptoms.*

My doctor was keen for me not to take antibiotics, so I was trying to fight this as hard as I could without medication. But my immune system struggled to cope, and the result was my joints became stiff and my neck, ankles, knees, hands and wrists became severely swollen and very painful. How was I to continue to perform?

Despite several visits to Harley Street doctors and numerous blood tests, no one seemed to be able to tell me what was wrong. Not knowing was very worrying and having to continue with the show which involved a considerable amount of dancing made it twice as bad.

The press representative on Anything Goes *having been a lupus sufferer herself recognised some of my symptoms, and she suggested an appointment with Dr Graham Hughes at St Thomas' Hospital, the leading consultant in this field. Due to his diagnosis a course of medication was prescribed which put me back on track and enabled me to carry on performing.*

After a year of treatment I was well again and have been ever since except for a mild recurrence in 2001 from a flu jab that triggered another reaction in my immune system. However, once diagnosed it was under control immediately.

I suffered on both occasions from mis-diagnosis. Ensuring doctors recognise symptoms seems to be the key to future care for sufferers of lupus. Knowing one's own body and reading the signs is also very important.

If we are to help people in the future who suffer from the severe forms of this disease then we need to build further awareness in this country amongst the medical profession as well as with the general public.

Chapter 14

What the Future Holds

Forecasting the future when it comes to lupus is as haphazard as predicting the weather in Britain. Will there be a cure for lupus in the next twenty years or so? Will we know what causes this disease? Will there be a 'magic bullet' that will bring the hooligan immune system back in line? There are no conclusive answers to these pressing questions – only educated guesses. To understand how far we could progress in the future it is relevant to summarise how far we have come in a short space of time.

The world map of lupus back in the 1960s was very different from how it is today. Large parts of the globe, like the Antipodes, China, Africa and South America, were not represented because lupus wasn't recognised there. Many medical departments, including rheumatology, considered lupus to be a small-print esoteric disease. A medical mythology had developed that said lupus was a killer disease and pregnancy was forbidden if you had it. As we have seen in this book, all these factors have changed beyond recognition in the past few decades. Lupus clinics have opened up worldwide, and there are now strong links between specialists internationally. Information is shared, and that pooling of resources speeds up advances in this field.

The number of people with lupus will continue to grow as a new generation of general practitioners becomes acquainted with the disease. The recognition of subsets such as Hughes syndrome and Sjogren's syndrome will contribute to this growth. It is likely that lupus and Hughes syndrome will become recognised as the most common autoimmune diseases.

Most of the gaps on the world map have now been filled. Look at Africa, for instance. It is still the general perception that lupus is not common there, but greater knowledge and improved diagnostic techniques have resulted in a steep rise in numbers. It could be that in the next few years we will realise that lupus is just as common on this continent at it is in Europe and the Americas. Having said that, there do seem to be genuine geographic differences in how prevalent the disease is. As has been said earlier (*see page 158*) there is a much higher incidence of lupus among Afro-Caribbean and Afro-American populations. Hughes syndrome is also found in greater numbers among Arabic populations.

Genetics

The mapping of the genome has had an impact on every aspect of medicine. Lupus is no exception. Clinicians have always known that lupus has a genetic component. Patients have also had their suspicions when they have looked at their family medical histories and recognised that lupus might have been present in past generations but not diagnosed.

Nearly thirty years ago, Dr Hughes and his team at the Hammersmith Hospital, working with Doctors Fielder and

Batchelor in the department of immunology, first reported an association with a genetic abnormality in the protein called 'complement'. Although to date there are few genetic studies of lupus, we do know that a lot of work is in the pipeline and it doesn't take too much imagination to predict that soon scientists will define the links between lupus and specific areas of the genetic ticker-tape. There is a word of caution here, however. Although for most major diseases the identification of a genetic marker does advance our understanding, it does not necessarily improve treatment.

Blood tests

There will be an expansion in the science of blood tests (*see also page 69*). Already these have revolutionised lupus, in particular the anti-DNA test for classical lupus, the anti-ENA test for certain lupus sub-groups, such as Sjogren's syndrome and subcutaneous lupus, and the antiphospholipid antibodies test for Hughes syndrome. The tests are constantly being honed and refined. New tests are under scrutiny; they might not be 'headline' developments, but they are nonetheless vital to the more precise diagnosis and management of patients.

At the moment having to have a biopsy – whether it is for the kidneys, skin, ovaries or brain – is at best uncomfortable and at worst painful and traumatic. With the work that is under way, in the foreseeable future these tests will be used less and less and will be replaced by testing through having blood taken from a simple finger prick. Some tests will no longer need blood samples but will be done using saliva, and people will be able to buy the kits themselves and do the tests at home, saving time and money.

Drug treatment – new and old

There is a race among laboratories and pharmaceutical companies around the world to come up with the next generation of designer drugs to combat lupus. There hasn't been a new 'drug' as such in the past forty years, so there is a desperate need for progress in this field.

Many of the drugs are based on knowledge of the way immune cells and antibodies lock together with the body's own cells. For example, we know reasonably precisely how certain antibodies link up with cell membranes – such as blood vessel membranes – in Hughes syndrome. To develop an agent that could precisely interfere with or even block this interaction would be real progress. It would be like finding a 'magic bullet' targeting the local conflict. Unlike the conventional immunosuppressive drugs, which act more like an atom bomb by affecting both good and bad cells, these medications would go straight to the problem, do their job and leave the rest of the body in peace.

The armoury of drugs used in lupus has always been restricted. The list is brief – antimalarials, steroids, aspirin, anti-coagulants, NSAIDs and immunosuppressives. The up side of this is that these medications have stood the test of time. 'Advances' have been made with all of them, enabling them to be used more effectively. The doses for many of them can now be tailored to limit side effects, which is particularly valuable in the case of steroids because of their strong side effects. The championing of more conservative regimes for steroids and cyclophosphamide has been a crucial step forward.

With the more toxic immunosuppressive drugs there are promising new agents such as Mofetyl. This drug is proving to do the job well with fewer side effects, and is rapidly becoming widely used as a preferred treatment in this category.

Over the next few decades, as there is a greater awareness of lupus so the pressure will grow for governments and governmental organisations to put funding in place to carry out the research that is so badly needed. We have already seen a surge in public interest and support for issues relating to SLE. A key thing to bear in mind about lupus is that if we can pin down the cause and possibly even a cure, then it will be like dropping a stone into a still pool. The reverberations will be felt right across the medical world because understanding lupus will mean having a greater knowledge about autoimmunity in general, so it will bring us closer to sorting out HIV, MS, ME and so on.

Dr Bob Lahita in New Jersey has a dream that one day there will be a hospital dedicated not just to lupus but also to all autoimmune conditions, allowing them all to be dealt with under one roof. This makes sense. After all, our immune system can be our best friend or our worst enemy. Getting some control over it will make all the difference.

Glossary of Medical Terms

acute a condition that comes on quickly and for a short duration.

adrenal glands small organs located above the kidneys, which produce steroid hormones.

aetiology the cause of an illness.

alopecia hair loss.

analgesic a painkilling drug.

anaemia a low red blood cell count.

antibodies proteins made by white blood cells that defend against bacteria and other foreign bodies.

anticoagulant drug that thins the blood.

antigen a protein that stimulates the formation of antibodies.

anti-inflammatory an agent that suppresses inflammation.

antinuclear antibodies (ANA) proteins in the blood that react with the nuclei of cells.

antiphospholipid antibodies antibodies that can make the blood more inclined to clot.

autoimmune disease a 'self-allergy', where the immune system attacks part or parts of the body that are otherwise healthy.

B-cell one of the groups of immune cells (lymphocytes).

biopsy a diagnostic procedure involving the removal of a small sliver of tissue that is then examined under a microscope.

butterfly rash a hallmark symptom of lupus, where there are red markings across the nose and cheeks that can appear in a wing shape.

chronic an illness that persists over a long period of time.

CNS central nervous system.

complement a series of proteins that play a part in immune defences.

connective tissue the substance that holds the muscle, skin and joints together.

cutaneous something that relates to the skin.

dermatomyositis inflammation of the muscle due to an autoimmune process; it can include skin rashes.

diuretics medication that increases the secretion of fluids.

DNA deoxyribonucleic acid, the chemicals in the cell nucleus that carry the genetic code, the building blocks of the body.

endocarditis inflammation of the inside wall of the heart.

enzyme a protein that speeds up chemical reactions in the body.

erythema a reddish colour.

flare the onset of disease activity, when symptoms become exacerbated.

haemoglobin the protein in red cells responsible for carrying oxygen around the body.

hydrotherapy physiotherapy in water.

immunity the body's defence against foreign substances.

immunosuppressives drugs used to cut down immune responses.

livedo reticularis a blotchy discolouration of blood vessels often found on the wrists and knees.

lymphocyte a type of white blood cell that is part of the immune system.

lymphatic system a network of glands that are strategically placed around the body to act as a first line of defence against the spread of infection.

macrophage a type of white blood cell that works in conjunction with lymphocytes to kill foreign material.

MRI magnetic resonance imaging, a type of scan that uses magnetism rather than X-rays.

nephritis inflammation of the kidneys.

neuropathy disease of the nerves.

neurological to do with brain function.

nucleus centre of a cell that contains the DNA.

obstetrician a specialist in pregnancy.

orthopaedic surgeon a doctor who deals with musculo-skeletal structures.

osteoporosis thinning of bone.

pathogenic causing disease or abnormal reactions.

pathology abnormal cellular or anatomical features.

pericarditis inflammation of the delicate tissue membrane surrounding the heart.

pericardium membrane around the heart.

photosensitivity sensitivity to ultraviolet (UV) light, especially from the sun.

plasma the fluid portion of the blood.

platelet a component of blood responsible for clotting.

pleurisy inflammation of the pleura, which is the delicate lining of the lungs.

protein a collection of amino acids.

proteinuria excess protein levels in the urine.

psoriasis chronic skin disorder.

psychosis serious mental illness, involving loss of contact from reality.

puerperium the period of time soon after giving birth.

pulse steroids high doses of steroids given intravenously over one to three days.

purpura red spots under the skin.

remission period of time free of disease.

rheumatoid arthritis chronic disease of the joints.

rhinitis inflammation in the nose.

sclera whites of the eyes.

scleritis inflammation in the whites of the eyes.

Septrin an antibiotic that can trigger a lupus flare.

steroids a shortened term for corticosteroids, which are anti-inflammatory hormones produced by the adrenal gland or made synthetically

systemic affecting more than one part of the body.

T-cell one of the groups of immune cells (lymphocytes).

thrombocytopenia low platelet count.

thrombosis blood clot.

tinnitus ringing in the ears.

urinalysis analysis of urine.

vasculitis inflammation of the blood vessels.

Resources

UK contacts

LUPUS UK
www.lupusuk.com

Hughes Syndrome Foundation
www.hughes-syndrome.org.uk

St Thomas' Hospital Lupus Trust
www.lupus.org.uk

Lancashire/Cheshire Group
www.uklupus.co.uk

West Midlands Group
www.westmidlandslupus.co.uk

AntiCoagulation Europe
www.anticoagulation.org.uk

British Dermatological Nursing Group
www.bdng.org.uk

Worldwide contacts

American College of Rheumatology
www.rheumatology.org

Arthritis Foundation of America
www.arthritis.org

Hamline University, Minnesota
www.hamline.edu/lupus

Lupus Foundation of America
www.lupus.org

Lupus Canada
www.lupuscanada.org

The SLE Foundation
www.lupusny.org

Lupus Research Institute
www.lupusresearch.org

Lupus Trust of New Zealand
www.lupus.org.nz

Lupus Association of Singapore
http://home1.pacific.net.sgl–lupusas

Lupus Australia Queensland Inc
www.lupus.com.au

Lupus Australia Foundation
www.lupusvic.org.au

Lupus Association of New South Wales
www.lupusnsw.org.au

Lupus Association of Tasmania
www.hotkey.net.au/-lupustas

Index